- An estimated eight million people in the United States have diabetes and do not know it
- ''An onion a day'' increases the action of insulin
- Eating meat can cause sugar cravings
- When to administer insulin for optimal blood glucose control
- With the McDougall Diet Program, seventy-five percent of Type II diabetics can stop taking insulin, and more than ninety-five percent can stop taking all hypoglycemic pills
- Drinking red raspberry tea promotes insulin production

PLUS HERBAL REMEDIES FOR OPTIMAL
PHYSICAL HEALTH, MOVEMENT THERAPY FOR
GOOD CIRCULATION, BIOENERGY THERAPIES
SUCH AS ACUPRESSURE FOR STRENGTH
AND ENERGY, AND OXYGEN THERAPY TO
SPEED HEALING

THE DELL NATURAL MEDICINE LIBRARY

PREVENTION, HEALING, SYMPTOM RELIEF . . .
FROM NATURE TO YOU

THE DELL
NATURAL MEDICINE LIBRARY

NATURAL MEDICINE
FOR DIABETES

Deborah R. Mitchell

Foreword by Gabriel Cousens, M.D.

A Lynn Sonberg Book

A Dell Book

Published by
Dell Publishing
a division of
Bantam Doubleday Dell Publishing Group, Inc.
1540 Broadway
New York, New York 10036

IMPORTANT NOTE: Neither this nor any other book should be used as a substitute for professional medical care or treatment. All readers should seek the guidance of a physician or other qualified health practitioner before implementing any of the approaches to health suggested in this book. Also, please note that research about natural approaches to managing diabetes is ongoing and subject to interpretation. Although all reasonable efforts have been made to include the most up-to-date and accurate information in this book, there can be no guarantee that what we know about this complex subject won't change with time. All rights reserved.

Published by arrangement with Lynn Sonberg Book Associates
10 West 86th Street
New York, NY 10024

Illustrations by Jackie Aher

Printed in the United States of America

Published simultaneously in Canada

July 1997

10   9   8   7   6   5   4

OPM

CONTENTS

PART III: MEDICAL THERAPY FOR DIABETES

FOREWORD

Natural Medicine for Diabetes offers options for managing diabetes that you may not have encountered before. The information in this book has been carefully researched; yet even as you read this page, what we know about diabetes, its complications, and how both natural and conventional medicine fit into the diabetes management picture is growing and changing. In my experience as a holistic physician over the past twenty-five years, this book is a guide for growth and change toward a better and better life with diabetes.

The natural therapies discussed in this book address four key areas: nutrition, exercise, stress reduction, and the mind/body connection. All of the healing approaches are meant to complement your current diabetes management programs. More important, they will help you take more control of your health. They will not cure diabetes; but they will make your life with it fuller, more relaxed, more balanced, and, hopefully, less challenged with diabetic complications. Natural medicine can do all this . . . but only if you take the first step to add it to your life and make the commitment to keep it there.

Conventional (allopathic) medicine plays an important role in many cases of diabetes, especially if you are insulin-dependent. Yet the majority of people with diabetes in the United States have the non–insulin variety—and most of them are nonetheless taking insulin, diabetic pills, or both to control their disease. With a holistic approach there is no need for this.

People who have a chronic condition such as diabetes are often fraught with fears, anger, frustration, and depression. They are afraid of having insulin reactions, angry about having diabetes, frustrated about limitations on their lifestyle, and depressed overall about their condition. Most of all, they often feel helpless and trapped: they are overweight, taking pills, injecting insulin, worried about their feet and their eyes and their sex life and their heart. . . . They are out of touch with themselves. And good management and control of diabetes requires that people be willing to be in touch with their body and their emotions, and to make the changes necessary to be free of the idea of diabetes as a chronic condition.

Natural Medicine for Diabetes helps you with both. In Part I, you get answers to questions that can prepare you to make the mind/body connection, questions such as: What is diabetes? Who do I turn to for help? How can I manage concerns such as monitoring glucose levels, eating out, traveling, and insulin reactions? What role do emotions play in diabetes? Part II builds on this foundation by introducing you to natural ways to get in touch with your physical body and your emotional/spiritual self and by showing you how to bridge the gap that may be keeping you from a more vital, complete life with diabetes.

Natural Medicine for Diabetes is a reliable resource for you and anyone who is dealing with diabetes. Whether you choose to complement your conventional management program with one or more of the natural approaches explained in this book or use the resources listed in the back to explore further, always see your physician and management team first to discuss your choices and options. Diabetes can be managed safely and naturally when you are ready to take control. It is amazing how much people can get freed from the diabetic lifestyle and complications when they are willing to make the holistic changes in their life to do so. This book is wonderful in the way it gives you the tools to make your life significantly freer from diabetes.

GABRIEL COUSENS, M.D.,
Director of Tree of Life Rejuvenation Center
and author of *Conscious Eating*
February 1997

INTRODUCTION

This book explores some of the safest and most effective natural therapies for the control and management of diabetes. Researchers in fields as diverse as endocrinology, herbal medicine, exercise physiology, pharmacology, and mind/body medicine are making new discoveries nearly every day about the mechanics of diabetes and the benefits of using natural medicine approaches to treat, control, and manage this disease. These therapies do not pretend or claim to cure diabetes: they are offered as safe, natural therapeutic options to complement your current management program. If you take insulin now, you should of course continue to take it, but you and your doctor may find that your insulin needs decrease when you try some of the approaches in this book. In most if not all cases, we believe you will enjoy less stress, better health, and improved emotional well-being by using the natural therapies presented here. These natural approaches allow you to more fully experience how diabetes affects your body so you can take better control of your disease without it taking control of you. This book is for you and anyone with diabetes who wants to try new, natural approaches to control and manage their condition. It is for individuals with diabetes who resolve to live as fully, naturally, and drug free as possible.

The natural therapies offered in this book are part of a holistic, complementary approach to health. Unlike drugs, you can generally try several natural healing techniques at the same time, such as meditation, nutritional supplementation, and yoga, without suffering adverse effects. In any case, always consult with your physician before you start any new therapeutic approach, natural or otherwise, monitor your progress, and keep your physician and other health practitioners apprised of the healing approaches you are using.

Natural Approach to Diabetic Care

The general rule to remember while you read this book is this: Among people with diabetes, the key to good health and to preventing and reducing the risk of diabetic complications is to achieve and maintain optimal blood glucose levels. The natural therapies presented here are designed to help you achieve that goal. You can have more control over your diabetes and your overall health. This book looks at natural healing approaches to diabetes in the following areas:

• Nutritional supplementation and herbal remedies allow you to provide optimal nourishment for your physical body and gain better control of your physical health.

• Movement therapy provides you with enjoyable ways to keep your body strong and flexible, control your blood glucose levels, and maintain good circulation.

• Bioenergy therapies, such as acupressure, acupuncture, biomagnetics, homeopathy, polarity therapy, reflexology, and tai chi help build a stronger, more vital life energy.

• Mind/body therapies, such as breathing, hypnosis, massage, meditation, visualization and guided imagery, and yoga help you manage the everyday stress of having diabetes, and good management helps you maintain a good blood glucose level. They also can prepare you for times of crisis, such as the beginning signs of a major diabetic complication, and help you better cope with the challenges diabetes presents.

• Oxygen therapy, considered by some to be an "alternative" medical therapy and by others to be a natural therapy, is reserved for treatment of poor wound healing.

How This Book Can Help You

Diabetes is a chronic disorder. These pages do not contain a magic potion to make it go away. They do, however, contain hope, answers, and tools to help you take control of your disease. Nearly half of the 16 million people with diabetes in the United States have not been formally diagnosed with the disease, yet many suspect they have it. Whether you think you have diabetes or you have been diagnosed with the disease, you will want to turn to Part I of this book, in which we explain the signs and symptoms of diabetes, how the disease affects the body, and the complications that are often associated with diabetes. We talk about both the natural and conventional health practitioners you can turn to for help and what to expect from them. We look at the intricate connection between the mind and body and how understanding and nurturing that relationship can help you manage your diabetes.

In Part II, we present the most effective natural healing methods to treat diabetes: acupressure, acupuncture, biofeedback, bio-Magnetic Touch Healing, breathing therapy, herbal medicine, homeopathy, hypnosis, massage, meditation, movement therapy, nutrition, nutritional supplements, oxygen therapy, polarity therapy, reflexology, tai chi, visualization and guided imagery, and yoga. In each case we talk about how you can use this therapy yourself or whether you need a professional practitioner to help you; the benefits of the therapy and what it can do for you; and where to get additional help.

In Part III, we briefly discuss the current medical therapy for diabetes and the procedures for complications related to diabetes. Last are your information resources: a glossary; names and addresses of organizations and resources for therapies and practitioners discussed in the book, sources for herbs and homeopathic remedies, instructional videos and cassettes, and other products; and an extensive reading list.

One out of twenty people in the United States has diabetes. This book is for you and for them: to help all of you become aware of and better informed about natural therapies for diabetes. It is not intended to take the place of medication or medical advice from any health-care professionals. Complementary medicine does not replace traditional biomedicine; rather, it broadens the therapeutic possibilities. We offer you the opportunity to better control and manage diabetes and help prevent the complications associated with this disease in ways most other books on diabetes do not address.

NOTE: Diabetes is a serious, life-threatening disease. Do not attempt to self-diagnose or self-treat; always consult a physician, your health-care team, or both, before you try any type of therapy. The therapies offered in this book may be potentially helpful to you; however, always use them under the supervision of a qualified medical practitioner. If you have more than one health-care professional assisting you, keep each informed about the activities, medications, and therapies you are involved in.

PART ONE

YOU AND DIABETES

CHAPTER ONE

Understanding Diabetes

Each and every day, approximately 1,700 people in the United States are diagnosed with diabetes. Over the course of a year, that equals about 625,000 people who discover they have this chronic disease. The latest report (1995) from the National Institute of Diabetes and Digestive and Kidney Diseases (NIDDK) shows an estimated 16 million people in the United States with diabetes. Chances are that you've picked up this book because you or someone close to you is included in this figure.

In addition to its effects on personal health, diabetes is a financial burden. The NIDDK estimates that $92 billion is spent on diabetes each year: $45 billion in direct medical costs (costs directly attributable to diabetes) and $47 billion in indirect costs (disability, premature death, and work loss). Thus overall, diabetes has a major impact on individual lives and on society. To better understand the many facets of this disease, in this chapter we answer some basic questions about diabetes.

- What is diabetes?
- What are the different types?
- What are the risk factors?
- Which complications are associated with it?

We hope the answers to these questions will help you do two things: make management of your diabetes easier for you or for someone close to you; and serve as a stepping-stone to the natural healing therapies discussed in Part II of this book.

What Is Diabetes?

Diabetes mellitus—the scientific name for this disease—is a chronic disorder in which your cells cannot properly use the sugar, or glucose, your body obtains from the food you eat. To help your cells use glucose, they need a hormone called **insulin,** which allows your cells to accept and take in **glucose** (a simple sugar in the bloodstream that comes from the carbohydrates you eat) to use as energy. In people who do not have diabetes, the **pancreas**—a small organ behind the stomach (see Figure I-1)—secretes the proper amount of insulin to meet the cells' needs. In people with diabetes, this process goes awry, and the amount of glucose in the blood, or the **blood glucose level,** can rise dangerously. Individuals who do not produce any insulin have Type I, or insulin-dependent, diabetes. Those who have low insulin production, or whose cells are not sensitive to insulin and so do not accept it, have Type II, or non–insulin-dependent, diabetes.

To understand why insulin is important in diabetes, you need to understand how your metabolism works. Briefly, your body derives energy from three sources in the food you eat: glucose from carbohydrates, fatty acids from fats,

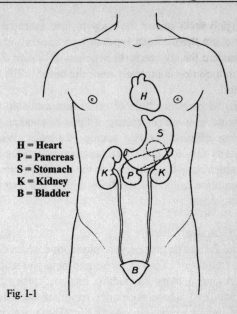

H = Heart
P = Pancreas
S = Stomach
K = Kidney
B = Bladder

Fig. I-1

and amino acids from protein. Glucose is the body's first choice for energy, protein is second, and fats are the least efficient and used as a last resort. Glucose is quickly absorbed into the bloodstream and heads for the cells so it can enter and supply them with energy. Extra glucose is stored in the liver and muscles until they are filled to capacity, and then the rest is stored in fat cells. If you have little or no insulin, however, or if your cells resist letting the sugar in, the glucose accumulates in the blood and causes **hyperglycemia**—a high level of glucose in the blood.

As glucose-rich blood passes through the kidneys, some glucose is retrieved. The excess glucose is eliminated in the urine (this condition is called **glycosuria**) and signals your body to pump more fluids through the kidneys to help eliminate the extra sugar. This action explains why diabetes is characterized by excessive thirst and urination. Excess urination (**polyuria**) causes the body to lose essential fluids, such as electrolytes, which are dissolved minerals and other compounds the body needs. In people with severe diabetes, urination may stop completely once the body's cells lose all their fluid.

When the body has little or no insulin available to help the cells get glucose for energy, it turns to another, though much less efficient, energy source—fat cells. When the body burns fats for fuel, it creates byproducts called ketones, which raise the acid level in the blood. The result is a toxic condition called **ketoacidosis,** which, if left untreated, can cause death.

Blood Glucose Levels

Several factors determine your blood glucose levels, such as diet, amount of exercise, stress and how you manage it, and hormone activity (including insulin, corticosteroids, and adrenaline). These hormones stimulate the release of glucose and its entry into your cells. These activities, in turn, either raise or lower your blood glucose levels. How well your body can regulate these levels can be determined by a **glucose tolerance test,** which is discussed in Chapter 3.

The normal range for blood glucose is about 60 mg/dL to 140 mg/dL (milligrams of glucose per deciliter of blood), depending on when you last ate. A level of 50 mg/dL is normal in people who are fasting, but levels lower than 45 mg/dL usually indicate hypoglycemia. Hypoglycemia and its symptoms are discussed later in this chapter.

Why Control of Diabetes Is Important

For many years, medical experts have believed that good control of blood glucose levels can reduce or eliminate the sudden complications of Type I diabetes (hypoglycemia, also known as insulin reaction or low blood glucose; and ketoacidosis) and may help reduce the risks of long-term problems such as stroke and eye and kidney complications in both Type I and II diabetes. Results of the DCCT (Diabetes Control and Complications Trial), a study conducted from 1983 to 1993 by the NIDDK, confirmed these ideas.

In this largest diabetes study ever carried out, data from 1,441 people with Type I diabetes showed that maintaining blood glucose levels as close to normal as possible slows the onset and progression of nerve, eye, and kidney diseases that accompany diabetes. Of particular interest is the finding that *any* sustained reduction in blood glucose levels, even in people with a history of poor glucose control, is beneficial.

The sooner you take control of your diabetes, the sooner you will enjoy better overall health and more peace of mind. Part II of this book offers you many natural, drug-free ways to achieve and maintain that control.

Types of Diabetes

Insulin is a key player in diabetes, and its role differs depending on the type of diabetes you have. There are two major types of diabetes—Type I and Type II—which we explain on pages 8–14 and refer to throughout the rest of this book. Two other types, gestational diabetes and secondary diabetes, are much less common and are explained briefly. All forms of diabetes can be treated with the natural healing methods described in this book.

TABLE I-1

COMPARISON OF TYPE I AND II DIABETES

	Insulin Dependent: I	**Non–insulin-Dependent: II**
Age of Onset	Usually before 20	Usually after 40
Insulin	Little or no insulin produced by pancreas	Insulin produced, but may be insufficient or can't be used
Cause	Heredity, infection, other factors	Inherited tendency, obesity, other factors
Symptoms	Obvious: extreme thirst, hunger; frequent urination, other factors	May not be obvious: fatigue, frequent thirst and urination
Onset	Sudden	Slow
Sex	M & F equal	F more
Weight	Majority thin	Majority overweight
Ketones	Found in urine	Usually none in urine
Treatment	Insulin, diet, exercise, self-management	Diet, exercise, self-management; oral insulin when necessary
Complications	Acute: insulin reactions, ketoacidosis Long-term: blood vessel problems in heart, brain, feet, eyes, nerves, and kidneys	Acute: usually none

Type I: Insulin-Dependent Diabetes

Insulin-dependent diabetes is sometimes called juvenile diabetes because it most often appears in childhood or adolescence. Symptoms are usually obvious and include excessive thirst and appetite, frequent urination, and fatigue. Children and adolescents who have these symptoms should be examined immediately by their physician (see Chapter 2 for diabetes testing). Some people also experience blurred vision, nausea, vomiting, abdominal pain, or rapid shallow breathing.

About 10 percent of all diabetics have Type I disease, and about thirty thousand new cases are diagnosed each year. The pancreas of individuals who have Type I diabetes produces little or no insulin because the **beta cells,** which manufacture insulin, have been totally or mostly destroyed. Exactly what causes the beta cells to be destroyed is uncertain. One popular explanation is that the body's immune system malfunctions and destroys them. Another is that a virus forces the body to create antibodies that instead destroy the beta cells. This theory is supported by recent research and is the subject of continuing investigation.

STAGES OF TYPE I DIABETES

Type I diabetes usually develops in four main stages: newly diagnosed, remission, intensification, and total diabetes. During the **newly diagnosed** stage, your body still produces some insulin, but it is not enough. You will probably need high doses of injected insulin until your blood glucose levels are brought close to normal levels. Once these levels are under control, your body may enter a **remission** stage, during which you will probably need small amounts of insulin daily. If you were to stop taking insulin, you could have an allergic reaction later when you reintroduce insulin to your body. The time during which your body loses its remaining ability to produce insulin is referred to as **intensification.** During this third stage, your need for injectable insulin increases. Once your pancreas has completely lost its ability to produce insulin, you have reached **total diabetes.** At this point, you and your management team will determine how, when, and what type of insulin injections you will need per day.

MANAGEMENT

People with Type I diabetes need to take insulin injections daily in order to stay alive; insulin cannot be taken by mouth because it is a protein and the acids in the stomach render the hormone ineffective. The insulin needs of people with Type I diabetes vary from person to person and are closely linked to their eating and exercise habits, management of stress, presence of infection, pregnancy, menstruation, and other factors. The types of insulin, their sources, and how they are administered are discussed in Part III of this book.

Based on the results of the DCCT, experts are now recommending the following treatment plan for Type I diabetes for selected individuals. The approach is referred to as "tight control" or intensive therapy, and requires that you:

- Test blood glucose levels four or more times a day
- Take four insulin injections daily or use an insulin pump
- Adjust your insulin doses based on your food intake and amount of exercise
- Strictly adhere to your eating and exercise programs
- Make monthly visits to your management team members, including your physician, nurse educator, dietitian, and mental health professional (latter individual as needed)

You and your physician can determine whether you are a candidate for tight control. Tight control is not recommended for people in the following categories:

- Children younger than thirteen years
- Elderly people
- Individuals with diabetic complications, such as end-

stage kidney disease, severe vision loss, coronary artery disease, or vascular disease
• People who experience hyperglycemia often

HEREDITY

Type I diabetes tends to run in families, although the association is not strong, as about 85 percent of people who develop Type I diabetes do not have an immediate family member with the disease. Risk factors for family members have been determined (see Table I-2).

TABLE I-2

If	Your Risk Factor
Your twin has diabetes	1 in 3
Your sibling has diabetes	1 in 14
One parent has diabetes	1 in 25
Your mother has diabetes	1 in 40–50
Your father has diabetes	1 in 20
No relative has diabetes	1 in 500

Adapted from: J. I. Rotter, et al. *Diabetes* 1983; 32:75A.

The general consensus among physicians is that people do not directly inherit Type I diabetes but rather a susceptibility to it. Researchers are looking for ways to detect diabetes before it becomes apparent, but as yet have not found a marker or indicator that is accurate and practical to use for testing purposes.

Type II Diabetes

It is estimated that 16 million people in the United States have Type II, or non–insulin-dependent diabetes mellitus. Approximately 90 percent of people with diabetes have this form of the disease. It is sometimes called adult-onset or maturity-onset diabetes because it usually appears in people older than forty years, although it can develop in people younger than twenty-five years.

Individuals with Type II diabetes produce their own insulin, but the body cannot use it properly. This problem may occur for various reasons. In some cases the insulin receptors on the outside of the cells do not accept the insulin, or there are too few receptors; for other people, the glucose enters the cells but the cells do not use it properly. These are examples of **insulin resistance,** in which the body resists the action of available insulin. Insulin resistance is caused by obesity and an inherited tendency for resistance. Although you can't change your genes, you can change your weight and eating habits, both of which can help you control your diabetes without drugs (see "Nutrition" in Part II). Not all people with Type II diabetes have insulin resistance; some produce too little insulin because they have too few beta cella. In less than 1 percent of people with Type II diabetes, a weak, ineffective form of insulin is produced. Regardless of the reason, the end result is the same: the cells do not get enough glucose.

SYMPTOMS

As Table I-1 shows, Type II diabetes differs from Type I in many ways. One problem with Type II diabetes is that it can be difficult to diagnose because it often produces only mild or no symptoms. Some people don't discover they have diabetes until they develop one or more of the complications associated with the disease (see "Diabetic Complications" pp. 20–31), or while they are undergoing a physical examination. Symptoms of Type II diabetes include the following:

- Fatigue
- Excessive thirst

- Frequent urination
- Sudden weight loss
- Blurred vision
- Slow wound healing
- Genital itching

If you have no symptoms and you feel all right, you may wonder why you should be concerned. Although people with Type II seldom experience the type of daily problems that can affect people with Type I disease, such as hypoglycemia or ketoacidosis, they often eventually develop long-term complications, such as neuropathy (nerve damage), heart disease, stroke, and circulation problems in their eyes, feet, and kidneys. These conditions usually develop slowly and are not detected until damage has occurred.

TRADITIONAL TREATMENT

People with Type II diabetes generally do not need to take insulin, yet according to the American Diabetes Association, about 30 percent of people with Type II do inject this drug daily. The safest and most preferred way to control and manage Type II diabetes, however, is weight control, diet, and exercise. Excess fat appears to hinder the body's sensitivity to insulin, and about 80 percent of people with Type II diabetes in Western countries are obese. Thus a commitment to weight loss and a healthy eating plan could eliminate the use of insulin in most people with Type II diabetes (see "Nutrition" in Part II).

Most people with Type II diabetes take oral hypoglycemic pills—or "diabetes pills"—at some point during their disease course to help overcome their resistance to insulin. These diabetes pills are not insulin, nor are they a substitute for diet and exercise management. They appear to stimulate the pancreas to release more insulin and may help increase the effectiveness of insulin once it reaches the cell receptor sites. Diabetes pills can be effective under the following conditions:

- For Type II diabetes only
- People older than age forty; occasionally for individuals in their thirties
- Presence of the disease for less than ten years
- Normal weight
- Have never taken insulin or never taken more than forty units per day

We discuss diabetes pills in more depth in Part III.

Gestational Diabetes

Between 2 and 5 percent of pregnant women develop gestational diabetes during their second or third trimester. Rates among African-Americans and Hispanics are higher, with the highest rate being among Native Americans (1 to 14 percent of pregnancies).

Gestational diabetes usually appears without symptoms, which is one reason why all pregnant women should be screened for diabetes between weeks twenty-four and twenty-eight of their pregnancy. At this stage of pregnancy, the placenta releases hormones that interfere with insulin. Women who cannot produce enough insulin to maintain normal blood glucose levels will develop gestational diabetes. Although gestational diabetes can be dangerous to both the fetus and the mother, the disease can be controlled through a strict diet. Improper or inadequate management can cause the child to take in too much glucose and grow abnormally large. These children then have a tendency to develop diabetes later in life.

The risk of getting gestational diabetes is increased in pregnant women who (1) have a family history of either Type I or II diabetes; (2) are older than thirty; (3) were overweight before becoming pregnant; (4) have ever had an elevated blood glucose level; and (5) had a previous pregnancy that ended in a stillbirth or a child weighing more than nine pounds. Prompt treatment usually results in a return to normal blood glucose levels after delivery. Within fifteen years, however, 60 percent of these women will develop diabetes.

Secondary Diabetes

Secondary diabetes is associated with conditions such as pancreatic disease, hormone disturbances, genetic syndromes, drug-induced diabetes, malnourishment, and insulin receptor abnormalities. Cases of secondary diabetes are uncommon and are not addressed separately in this book.

Risk Factors for Diabetes

Type I

The following are risk factors for Type I diabetes. They are guidelines only, as there is still much we do not know about diabetes.

AGE

The majority of cases appear before age twenty. In girls, the disease usually appears around twelve to thirteen years of age; among boys, it shows one to two years later. According to the NIDDK (1993), approximately 3.2 million adults age sixty-five years or older have Type I diabetes.

There may be a link between the mother's age at the time of her child's birth and the likelihood that child will develop Type I diabetes. Children with Type I diabetes are twice as likely to have been born to a woman older than age thirty-five. The reason for this fact is not known, although some researchers believe it is linked to the decline in glucose tolerance that occurs with age.

GENDER

Males and females have similar risk for Type I diabetes. Of the approximately 7.8 million people with either Type I or Type II diabetes, the NIDDK (1993) estimates that 4.2 million are women and 3.6 million are men.

RACE

Little research has been done in this area. Results from a few studies indicate that whites are 1.5 times more likely than blacks to have Type I diabetes. Children with British or Jewish backgrounds appear to have a 50 percent greater risk than those of Italian or French descent.

EXPOSURE TO VIRUSES

Several infections have been associated with the development of diabetes: German measles (rubella), mumps, infectious mononucleosis, infectious hepatitis, Coxsackie virus, and cytomegalovirus (a type of herpes that affects people who have an impaired or undeveloped immune system). It is believed these viruses may cause the autoimmune response to destroy a person's insulin-producing beta cells. In the case of German measles, the damage may occur even before the child is born: an infant infected with German measles while in the womb may have up to a 40 percent chance of developing Type I later in life.

IMPAIRED IMMUNE SYSTEM

For reasons still unknown to medical experts, 90 percent of children diagnosed with Type I diabetes have antibodies that have destroyed their beta cells. Whether the antibodies are produced to fight a virus, as mentioned above, or a genetic defect causes the body to create them, the result is the same: the immune system is compromised. As a result, people with Type I diabetes are at a greater risk of getting other autoimmune diseases, such as Addison's disease (a dysfunction of the adrenal gland), myasthenia gravis (weakness of certain muscles), pernicious anemia, and vitiligo (a loss of pigmentation of the skin).

HORMONES

Type I diabetes typically appears around the age of puberty, which leads many medical experts to believe growth hormones may play a role in triggering the disease. The pituitary gland secretes growth hormone, and the amount released can vary, depending on whether infection is present or a person is under stress. If excess growth hormone is released into the body, it can disrupt insulin's activity and may trigger Type I diabetes in individuals who are susceptible to the disease.

TOXINS, DRUGS, AND CHEMICALS

Many drugs have some impact on individuals predisposed to diabetes, although the full extent of the effect is not completely known. Steroids, for example, make the liver release glucose. Other drugs can raise blood glucose levels or disrupt the secretion of insulin. If you have a family history of diabetes and are taking any type of prescription or over-the-counter medications, talk with your physician about whether you should continue the medication.

Some experts believe that *N*-nitroso compounds such as streptozotocin, which are found in smoked and cured meats, destroy beta cells. Anecdotal evidence links dietary intake of *N*-nitroso compounds with diabetes in susceptible individuals.

AUTOIMMUNITY

Experts have found antibodies to pancreatic cells in 75 percent of people with Type I diabetes compared to 0.5 to 2 percent of people without diabetes. The high antibody levels decline progressively after the first few weeks the disease appears, which corresponds with the complete destruction of the beta cells.

COW'S MILK

Some experts have linked consumption of cow's milk to the development of Type I diabetes in children. They believe that drinking cow's milk during infancy may trigger Type I diabetes years later in children who are genetically susceptible to the disease. This controversial association is thought to occur in this way: certain proteins in cow's milk supply a foreign substance (an **antigen**) that tricks the child's immune system into destroying its own tissue—the beta cells in the pancreas. Research conducted at the Hospital for Sick Children in Toronto found antibodies, which indicate an immune reaction to milk proteins, in 100 percent of a group of children with Type I diabetes, but in only 2.5 percent of children without diabetes. Other studies show infants who are breast-fed and who are not given cow's milk until the second to third month of life are 40 percent less likely to develop diabetes by age fourteen than infants who are not breast-fed. Infants breast-fed until four months of age have a 50 percent lower risk of developing diabetes. (Also see "Gerson Therapy" under "Nutrition" in Part II.)

Type II

It is estimated that about 8 million people in the United States have Type II diabetes and do not know it. If after reading the following risk factors for Type II diabetes you believe you may have this condition, schedule an examination with your physician.

AGE

Most cases of Type II diabetes occur in adults age forty years and older. In the United States, about 20 percent of people age sixty-five years and older have diabetes.

HEREDITY

A family history of diabetes is a stronger risk factor in Type II diabetes than it is in Type I. Anyone who has family members with diabetes should be examined regularly for diabetes, especially after he or she reaches age forty. Studies of identical twins show that if one twin develops Type II diabetes before age thirty-five, the other twin has a 50 percent chance of getting the disease; after age forty, the chance is nearly 100 percent. If one parent has Type II diabetes, the children have a 35 percent chance of getting the disease later in life; if both parents have diabetes, the chance increases to 70 percent.

RACE

Because Type II diabetes has a tendency to be inherited, some groups have a higher incidence of the disease than others. The NIDDK has data on the percentage of adults with diabetes (diagnosed and undiagnosed) by race and ethnicity: Puerto Rican–Americans, 10.9 percent; African-Americans and Mexican-Americans: 9.6 percent; white Americans: 6.2 percent; Native Americans: 5 to 50 percent, depending on the nation. The Pima Indians in Arizona have the highest rate of diabetes in the world. Among Japanese-Americans, a study of second-generation Japanese-Americans forty-five to seventy-four years of age residing in King County, Washington, showed that 20 percent of the men and 16 percent of the women had diabetes.

OBESITY

Obesity can cause insulin resistance in people who have a genetic tendency to develop diabetes, prompting the disease to appear earlier than usual in some people. This occurs because fat "blocks" the insulin receptors on the cells. When glucose can't enter the cells, it builds up in the blood. Weight loss reduces the amount of fat and allows the cells to better utilize insulin by letting glucose in. Not all obese people get diabetes, however, probably because their pancreas produces enough insulin to control their blood glucose levels.

IMPAIRED GLUCOSE TOLERANCE

When blood glucose levels are higher than normal (between 140 and 199 mg/dL ninety minutes after a meal) but not high enough to be classified as diabetes, this is a condition known as impaired glucose tolerance, or IGT. This condition occurs in about 11 percent of adults and is a major risk factor for Type II diabetes. About 40 to 45 percent of persons age sixty-five years or older have either IGT or Type II diabetes.

CHROMIUM DEFICIENCY

Chromium levels appear to be a major factor in insulin sensitivity. This micronutrient acts as a cofactor in all insulin-regulating activities in the body. Chromium deficiency is common in the United States and can be corrected with supplementation (see "Nutritional Supplements" in Part II).

Diabetic Complications

People with Type I diabetes are especially susceptible to hypoglycemia and hyperglycemia (abnormally high blood glucose levels), although these conditions occasionally occur in people with Type II diabetes as well. Over time, either type of diabetes can damage the heart, blood vessels, kidneys, nerves, eyes, and teeth. Exactly how diabetes causes these problems is not clearly understood. Changes in the small blood vessels and nerves are common. Although scientists cannot predict who will develop complications, people who have had diabetes for many years are the most likely candidates.

Among people with undetected Type II diabetes, complications such as heart disease, stroke, kidney disease, vision problems, or nerve damage may be their first indication that they have diabetes. Skin infections, as well as infections of the kidneys, vagina, bladder, and gums, are common among people with diabetes, because bacteria that cause infections love sugar. If you have high blood glucose levels, you are more likely to develop problems. Thus early detection and treatment of diabetes, especially control of blood glucose levels, are essential in order to eliminate or reduce the occurrence of these conditions.

Next we discuss the major complications associated with diabetes. Many of the natural healing therapies in this book help prevent or treat these conditions.

Heart and Blood Vessel Disease

In heart disease, deposits of fat and cholesterol accumulate in the arteries that carry blood to the heart. Eventually, this buildup, called **atherosclerosis,** can block blood flow, and a potentially fatal heart attack can occur. Heart disease is the most common life-threatening disease associated with diabetes. The blood vessels of people with diabetes tend to harden more quickly than those of people without diabetes. According to the NIDDK (1993), cardiovascular disease is two to four times more common in people with diabetes and is a factor in 75 percent of diabetes-related deaths. Middle-aged people with diabetes have death rates twice as high and heart disease death rates about two to four times higher than middle-aged people without diabetes.

You can slow atherosclerosis by maintaining near normal blood glucose levels, following a low-fat diet, getting regular aerobic exercise, and enjoying therapies that promote blood circulation, such as massage, polarity therapy, tai chi, and yoga. Results of the Diabetes Complication and Control Trial show that tight control of blood glucose lowers the risk of developing high cholesterol, a cause of heart disease, by 35 percent.

Blocked and thickened blood vessels that supply blood to the brain can lead to stroke. Among people with diabetes, the risk of stroke is 2.5 times higher than in the general population. Another blood-vessel complication of diabetes is high blood pressure, or **hypertension.** High blood pressure affects 60 to 65 percent of people with diabetes and speeds up the process of atherosclerosis. The best preventive measures for blood vessel and heart problems include a low-fat, low-cholesterol, high-fiber diet; movement therapy; stress reduction techniques and overall body healing, such as biofeedback, biomagnetic touch healing, breathing therapy, hypnosis, massage (in some cases), meditation, tai chi, visualization, and yoga.

Foot Problems

Most people don't think about their feet until they hurt. People with diabetes, however, often don't know they are experiencing foot problems because diabetes can cause poor blood circulation or loss of feeling in the feet. Nerve damage, called **neuropathy,** is characterized by numbing, tingling, burning, loss of feeling, or pain, and many people with diabetes suffer from numbness in their feet. When an injury or other problem occurs, such as a cut, bruise, blister, or callus, people with diabetes may not be aware of it until infection sets in or other damage is done. Routine foot care (see Chapter 3) is essential to prevent foot damage.

Diabetes also causes narrowing and hardening of the blood vessels, which restricts circulation. When the feet don't get enough blood, the tissue not only has too much sugar, it also doesn't receive enough oxygen. Thus if you have a wound on your foot and blood flow is restricted, oxygen is also limited, healing cannot occur, and infection can set in. Once infected tissue kills the tissue surrounding it, gangrene can develop and may require amputation of toes, the foot, or lower leg. One way to treat poor wound healing is with oxygen therapy (see ''Oxygen Therapy'' in Part II).

Eye and Vision Problems

Diabetes can affect many parts of your eyes in several ways. Some of the effects go away once you get better control of your blood glucose levels. However, if you have had diabetes for many years, you may experience changes that threaten your vision. Changing levels of blood glucose, for example, can influence the balance of fluid in the lens of the eye, which in turn affects its focusing power. Blurred vision can be the result. Another cause of blurred vision in diabetes occurs because of damage to the nerves that control eyesight.

Cataract and glaucoma are two common eye diseases among people with diabetes. A **cataract** is a clouding of the normally clear lens of the eye. If cataracts are detected early enough, good blood glucose control may reverse the problem. Once vision becomes significantly impaired, however, surgery is the only effective treatment. **Glaucoma** is a condition in which pressure within the eye damages the optic nerve that transmits visual images to the brain. Several homeopathic remedies are useful for cataracts and glaucoma (see ''Homeopathy'' in Part II). Another eye problem occurs if nerve damage, or neuropathy (see pp. 26–27) occurs in the eye. Neuropathy of the eye can make the eye muscles weak and double vision can result.

Potentially the most serious eye problem caused by diabetes is **retinopathy.** This complication occurs when the tiny blood vessels that supply the retina, the inner lining of the back of the eye, leak fluid or blood and damage the cells of the eye. At least 60 percent of people with diabetes for fifteen years or more have some form of retinopathy. According to the National Eye Institute, diabetic retinopathy affects approximately 7 million people in the United States. Among people with Type I diabetes, one in twenty gets retinopathy; among those with Type II, one in fifteen contracts the condition. The NIDDK (1993) reports that diabetes is the leading cause of new cases of blindness among adults twenty to seventy-four years of age. From twelve thousand to twenty-four thousand new cases of blindness per year are caused by diabetic retinopathy. Poor glucose control, kidney disease, and hypertension all contribute to this malady; thus any natural therapy that treats these conditions can help prevent it. Laser surgery can seal leaking blood vessels and prevent loss of vision if caught in time (see Part III).

Kidney Disease

The kidneys are two organs located in front of the lowest ribs and near the spine. Their function is to filter waste products, such as creatinine and urea, from the blood, and to make urine. Tiny blood vessels in the kidneys called **glomeruli** perform these functions. Because diabetes causes blood vessels to narrow and harden, the glomeruli can become damaged, which in turn limits or destroys their ability to filter the blood.

Kidney disease is a serious problem among people with diabetes. If not detected early and treated promptly, it can cause kidney failure or death. Routine testing (see Chapter 2, "Other Tests") is essential in order to detect kidney disease, because symptoms related to kidney failure usually occur only when kidney function has dropped to less than 25 percent of normal capacity.

Kidney disease develops slowly; kidney failure usually begins fifteen to twenty years after people have been diagnosed with diabetes. About one third of people with Type I diabetes develop kidney disease. One early sign of the disease is the presence of protein, mostly in the form of **albumin,** in the urine. This condition is known as **proteinuria,** and it does not cause any symptoms, which is why a urine test for protein should be a routine part of your examinations. As the amount of albumin increases in the urine and decreases in the blood, water seeps out of the blood into the skin. The result is swelling of the legs and feet during the day (the result of being upright) and of the face and hands at night.

Damage to the glomeruli also causes **uremia,** which is characterized by the presence of the waste products urea and creatinine in the blood. These two products are also tested for during routine examinations. The first signs of uremia are nausea, loss of appetite, weakness, and vomiting.

High blood pressure can be both a cause and a result of kidney disease. As kidney disease proceeds, increased damage to the kidneys leads to high blood pressure. Also, people who already have high blood pressure when kidney disease is diagnosed run an even greater risk of kidney function loss. Thus early detection and treatment of even mild hypertension is critical for people with diabetes.

The stage at which the kidneys stop functioning is called **end-stage renal disease (ESRD).** Diabetes is the leading cause of ESRD, accounting for about 36 percent of all cases. End-stage kidney disease is the final stage of a slow deterioration of the kidneys, which is known as **nephropathy.** Approximately fifty thousand people have ESRD as a result of diabetes. In people with diabetes, both high blood pressure and high blood glucose levels increase the risk of developing ESRD. Heredity, diet, and other medical conditions are factors that can lead to nephropathy as well. Treatment for ESRD is either dialysis, which involves being attached to a machine that filters your blood and takes out the waste products; or transplantation of a healthy kidney.

Individuals with Type I diabetes are more likely to get ESRD than those with Type II. About 40 percent of people with Type I develop severe kidney disease and ESRD by the age of fifty. Blacks and Native Americans develop diabetes, nephropathy, and ESRD at rates higher than whites and Hispanics. Type II diabetes also causes 80 percent of the ESRD among these two groups. Experts have no explanation for these higher rates.

Kidney problems can be prevented or slowed significantly if you control your blood glucose levels, eat a low-protein, low-salt diet, and prevent high blood pressure. These recommendations are supported by the findings of the DCCT, which showed that tight blood glucose control can prevent the development and slow the progression of diabetic kidney disease by 50 percent.

Nerve Damage

Neuropathy, or nerve damage, is very common among people with diabetes. Nerves reach into every part of your body, thus any nerve damage has potentially far-reaching effects. Symptoms of neuropathy can range from burning pain and numbness of the feet, legs, or hands to dizziness upon standing to sexual problems such as impotence or vaginal dryness. The good news from the DCCT is that the risk of nerve damage is reduced by 60 percent in people who practice tight control.

Scientists have several explanations as to how diabetes causes neuropathy. One is that the small blood vessels that supply the nerves with nutrients and oxygen are damaged and prevent or hinder messages from getting through. Another idea is that diabetes destroys the fat coating around the nerves and distorts the messages. In any case, according to the NIDDK, about 60 to 70 percent of people with diabetes have mild to severe forms of diabetic nerve damage. One of the most common areas affected by diabetes is the stomach and intestines. Many people with diabetes have what is called "slow stomach" or **gastroparesis,** which means the stomach empties slowly and causes a feeling of fullness and may cause vomiting and nausea. Problems with the intestines can include diarrhea and constipation.

Neuropathy also can affect the nerves that go to the heart and blood vessels. Symptoms of this type of neuropathy include elevated pulse rate, irregular heartbeat, and dizziness or fainting upon standing from a sitting or reclining position.

If you experience "pins and needles," numbness, tingling, and/or burning in your hands, arms, feet, or legs, you may have **peripheral neuropathy.** These feelings can occur on one or both sides of the body. Numbness can be serious, especially in your feet, as it affects your ability to feel pain. Severe forms of diabetic nerve disease are a major factor in foot amputations. More than half of lower limb amputations (toes, feet, and lower leg) in the United States occur among people with diabetes; from 1989 to 1992, the average number of amputations performed each year among people with diabetes was fifty-four thousand.

Good blood glucose control and routine examination of your nervous system are the best preventive steps against neuropathy. Treatment of painful neuropathies include biofeedback, hypnosis, meditation, visualization, and medications.

Dental Disease

Periodontal disease, which can lead to tooth loss, occurs with greater frequency and severity in people with diabetes. Approximately 30 percent of people age nineteen years or older with Type I diabetes have periodontal disease. Among Pima Indians, who have the highest rate of Type II diabetes in the world, the rate of tooth loss is fifteen times higher than in other people with Type II diabetes, and the incidence of periodontal disease is 2.6 times higher. Good blood glucose control, proper daily dental care (see Chapter 3), and twice-yearly dental checkups can help prevent dental problems.

Hypoglycemia

Hypoglycemia—also called low blood sugar or insulin reaction—is a common condition among people with diabetes. It occurs when blood levels of glucose drop too low (below 70 mg/dL) to properly fuel the body. When you consume carbohydrates, the body's main dietary sources of glucose, the glucose enters the bloodstream and heads for the cells. Insulin and glucagon control the amount of glucose in the blood. If you do not carefully monitor your medication use, food intake, activity level, and alcohol use, you risk getting hypoglycemia (see Table I-3). Symptoms of hypoglycemia include weakness, hunger, drowsiness, confusion (e.g., you can't tell time or find things), dizziness, hand tremors, clumsiness, irritability, headache, inability to detect sweet tastes, blurred vision, restlessness, insomnia, rapid heartbeat, sweating, and a cold, clammy feeling. In severe cases, loss of consciousness or coma can occur.

Hypoglycemia occurs most often in people with Type I diabetes and in some with Type II diabetes who use insulin. People with Type II diabetes who take oral diabetes drugs also are susceptible to hypoglycemia. Good blood glucose control is the primary way to prevent hypoglycemia. If you think you are having an insulin reaction, check your blood glucose level. If it is below 70 mg/dL, counteract the reaction by eating fifteen grams of carbohydrates, such as four ounces of fruit juice, two tablespoons of raisins, several glucose tablets, or two large sugar cubes.

If hypoglycemia is not treated with glucose and the stress hormones do not increase the blood glucose level, severe hypoglycemia may result. Symptoms include confusion, convulsions, strange behavior, and loss of consciousness. People with these reactions need to be treated by someone who can inject a substance called **glucagon,** a hormone that raises blood glucose levels (see Part III).

TABLE I-3
CAUSES AND SYMPTOMS OF
HYPERGLYCEMIA AND HYPOGLYCEMIA

CAUSES

Hyperglycemia (too much blood glucose)	Hypoglycemia (too little blood glucose)
Too little or poorly timed oral meds	Too much or poorly timed insulin or pills
Too much food, esp. sweets, or poorly timed meals	Missed meals, too little food or poorly timed
Illness: fever, colds, flu, surgery	More exercise than usual or poorly timed exercise
Emotional stress	Emotional stress
Bad medicines (out of date, etc.)	Use of alcohol in empty stomach
Less exercise than usual	

SYMPTOMS

Hyperglycemia	Hypoglycemia
Unusual thirst	Shaky, dizzy, weak
Frequent urination	Irritable
Fatigue, extreme tiredness	Pounding heart
Vision changes	Hunger, nervousness, headache
Persistent infections	Numbness or tingling (fingers,
Nausea and vomiting	lips)
Deep, rapid breathing	Blurred or double vision
Fruity breath	Slurred speech, confused
High urine ketone levels	thinking
	Seizures, night sweats
	Restless sleep, sweats
	Unconsciousness

Hyperglycemia

The opposite of low blood glucose is high blood glucose, or hyperglycemia. This condition can lead to ketoacidosis, which develops when there is insufficient insulin in the blood to allow glucose to be used by the cells for energy. The body then uses the fat cells for its energy. Because fats cannot be adequately broken down, ketones are formed and can build up in the blood. Without enough insulin in the blood, the ketones are filtered into the urine, where large amounts can result in ketoacidosis. Left untreated, ketoacidosis can result in coma or death.

Symptoms of ketoacidosis include dry mouth and abdominal pain. Left untreated with insulin and fluids, nausea, vomiting, heavy breathing, and loss of consciousness occur, and eventually, death. Hyperglycemia can be prevented if you maintain good blood glucose control and you test your urine for ketones whenever your blood glucose is 240 mg/dL or higher, you feel ill, you have been under great stress, or whenever your management team believes it is necessary.

Sexual Problems

Both men and women can experience sexual problems associated with diabetes. Among men, impotence (an inability to achieve and maintain an erection sufficient for vaginal penetration) is the most common diabetes-related sexual problem, followed by retrograde ejaculation (inability to ejaculate even though orgasm occurs); among women, poor lubrication and/or difficulty reaching orgasm are reported most often. All of these sexual problems can be associated with nerve damage in people with diabetes. Sometimes, however, sexual difficulties are psychological and are related to anxiety and stress about having diabetes and about how your partner may feel about you having the disease.

If you are experiencing sexual problems, it is recommended that you and your partner consult your mental health practitioner to help you deal with the issue. If your sexual problems are caused by nerve damage or low hormone levels, medical treatments such as penile implants, hormone injections, and drug therapy are available. Discuss these options with your health-care team.

In this chapter we have given you a broad overview of what diabetes is all about so you can be better prepared to meet the challenges it gives you. In the next chapter you will come face-to-face with diabetes and some of the individuals in both conventional and natural medicine who can help you meet those challenges.

CHAPTER TWO

Where Do I Turn for Help?

Perhaps you have already been diagnosed with diabetes. Maybe you suspect you have diabetes but are not sure. Or perhaps you have family members, relatives, or friends who have been wondering whether they have diabetes. After all, medical experts believe that for every case of diabetes that is diagnosed, another one is undiagnosed: in the United States, that means 16 million people have the disease, but only 8 million are formally diagnosed. Could you or someone you know be among the undiagnosed?

This chapter begins with an explanation of "Signs of Diabetes." These signs, which expand on those listed in Chapter 1, are offered as guidelines for you and others who are in the "not sure" and "wondering" groups mentioned above. If you think you may have diabetes, see your physician as soon as possible for an examination. Do not self-diagnose or self-treat without the supervision of a physician.

Say you've read the signs of diabetes and decide to make an appointment for an examination and consultation. Who should you call? What can you expect during your visit? What kind of tests will be conducted? If diabetes is diagnosed, who, in addition to your primary physician, will be involved in the management of your disease? Which natural therapy practitioners can offer you healing techniques that will complement conventional treatment?

This chapter offers answers to all of these questions. For more in-depth information not included here, ask your health practitioner. You also are referred to the appendices for names and phone numbers of organizations that can help you and to the Bibliography and Suggested Reading for additional reading.

Signs of Diabetes: Early Warnings

Some health problems that may signal diabetes can show up months or years before diabetes can be detected. This is true more often in cases of Type II than in Type I diabetes. Often these symptoms are mild, and you may dismiss them as just feeling "under the weather" or attribute them to the flu or stress. In Type I diabetes, however, symptoms of the disease usually come on quickly. If diabetes runs in your family and you are experiencing any of the early-warning signs listed below, please have an examination by your physician.

Skin Changes

Diabetes affects all the blood vessels. If the blood supply is hindered in any way, the skin may become very dry and itchy, especially in the genital and anal areas. You may experience skin infections, such as boils or abscesses, that are difficult to eliminate or will not heal. Lingering fungal or yeast infections, such as athlete's foot or candidiasis (a yeast infection that causes vaginal itching and a white discharge) may indicate diabetes in individuals with a family history of the disease.

Complications in Pregnancy

If you are pregnant and your blood sugar level is elevated, you may have **gestational diabetes,** which is discussed in Chapter 1. The appearance of gestational diabetes may be a warning of diabetes in the future. Other complications of pregnancy that may forewarn of diabetes include frequent miscarriages, toxemia (bacterial blood poisoning), a premature or difficult delivery, and a baby weighing more than nine pounds.

Frequent Urination and Extreme Thirst

In cases of diabetes, frequent urination frequently appears along with extreme thirst and, in children, bed-wetting. These symptoms are caused by high blood glucose levels. When there is too much glucose in the blood, the kidneys cannot process all of it and allow some of the excess sugar to be "dumped" into the urine, along with large amounts of water. As your body keeps getting rid of the excess glucose through urination, your body sends out signals that you are thirsty.

Constant Hunger

When your body cannot use the glucose circulating in your blood for energy, you get signals of hunger. Even though you may eat more, your body still can't use the glucose properly. Constant hunger is often accompanied by unusual and unexplained weight loss in people who have diabetes.

Leg Pains

Leg pains are caused by high blood glucose levels and are an early indication of nerve damage, called **neuropathy.** Neuropathy is discussed in Chapter 1.

Blurred Vision

When there is excess glucose in your blood, water is attracted to it. If you have high blood pressure, this can cause a buildup of fluids in your eyes, which results in distorted or blurred vision. Fortunately, your vision can return to normal once you begin treatment for diabetes.

Fatigue

This symptom can creep up on you. You may feel tired and sluggish for weeks, perhaps months, before you become concerned. The fatigue is the result of your body being unable to properly convert glucose into energy. Instead your body burns fat, which is an inefficient energy source, and causes weight loss.

Infections and Poor Wound Healing

High glucose levels cause your immune system to become less efficient, leaving you more susceptible to viruses and other infections, such as bladder and kidney infections, and especially vaginal infections among women. Cuts, bruises, blisters, boils, and surgical incisions that are slow to heal are also indications of a weakened immune system and a signal for diabetes.

Other Symptoms

Other signals of diabetes are less common and often go unnoticed or are thought to be associated with the flu or other medical conditions. These symptoms include nausea, vomiting, irritability, impotence, vaginal dryness, rapid shallow breathing, and abdominal pain.

Contacting a Physician

If you suspect you may have diabetes, an early diagnosis is best because it allows you to learn how to manage the condition and get on with your life. Most people make an appointment to see their primary-care physician—also referred to as a general or family practitioner, or an internist—who can order the tests necessary to confirm or negate your suspicions. If you get a diagnosis of diabetes, a team management approach is the recommended way to take care of your questions and needs (see "Health-Care Management Team Approach," pp. 39–40). You will not be left to deal with diabetes alone!

Diagnosing Diabetes

Both types I and II are diagnosed based on elevated blood glucose levels. The normal blood glucose levels range from 60 to 140 mg/dL immediately after eating. There are several tests your physician can order to determine your level.

If you go to a physician who does not already have your medical and personal history, both will be taken before testing begins. The glucose tolerance test (GTT) is the gold standard for diagnosing diabetes. This test involves eating a large amount of carbohydrates for three days, fasting the night of the third day, and then having blood drawn on the morning of the fourth day to measure the glucose level. You then drink a glucose solution and your blood is drawn again several times over a few hours to see how your body deals with glucose. Because this test takes several days, it is more often used when Type II diabetes is suspected.

If Type I diabetes is suspected, the doctor will likely choose to do a fasting blood glucose test in which a blood sample is drawn after an overnight fast. Glucose test results of more than 140 mg/dL after a fast or of 200 mg/dL or higher one to two hours after eating indicate diabetes.

Among people with newly diagnosed Type I diabetes, it is not unusual to see levels as high as 300 to 400 mg/dL.

The newest diagnostic method is the glycosylated hemoglobin test, also known as hemoglobin A1c (HgA1c). It measures the amount of glucose that attaches itself to the hemoglobin in your blood. This test has several advantages over other methods. Fasting is not necessary, and clinicians can read your average blood glucose levels over the past two to three months from a single blood sample. This test also helps determine the average of your glucose control over an eight-week period. As accuracy in reading these samples increases, this test is gaining in popularity.

After your physician has diagnosed probable diabetes using one test, she or he will confirm that suspicion by ordering another, different test. Thus if you originally had a fasting blood glucose test, your physician may follow up with a glycosylated hemoglobin test to rule out any variables that may have influenced the first results, such as illness, high stress, or a little "cheating" on your overnight fast.

Other Tests

Once diabetes has been diagnosed, you can expect to undergo several other tests then and during routine monitoring of your diabetes.

• *Urine Testing.* Several different tests of urine samples are done periodically to test for levels of protein, **creatinine,** and **microalbuminuria** (tiny amounts of the protein albumin in the urine). If protein appears in your urine, it means your kidneys are not filtering your blood adequately. This is one reason why a low-protein diet is recommended.

Your physician also will test for creatinine, a waste product of muscle activity. If creatinine builds up in the urine, it is a sign that your kidneys are not functioning properly.

A test for microalbuminuria detects very small amounts of protein in the urine. This test is an early warning sign for possible kidney damage. Early detection of microalbuminuria allows you to make the necessary dietary changes in protein intake to prevent kidney disease.

• *Cholesterol.* Your cholesterol levels will be tested periodically. Cholesterol is a waxlike substance that is manufactured by the body; it also enters the body in animal products such as meat and dairy products. Of the two types of cholesterol your body makes, the low-density lipoprotein (LDL) cholesterol deposits itself in your arteries while the high-density lipoprotein (HDL) cholesterol cleans up the LDL cholesterol and takes it to the liver for processing. The recommended level of HDL is 35 mg/dL or higher; for LDL, a level less than 130 mg/dL is ideal. To reduce your risk of heart and artery disease, limit your daily cholesterol intake to less than 300 mg, get sufficient exercise, and obtain the majority of your fat from unsaturated fats.

• *Triglycerides.* High levels of triglycerides—fats that circulate in the bloodstream—are associated with an increased risk of heart and blood-vessel disease in people with diabetes. To test for triglyceride levels, a blood sample will be tested after an overnight fast. High blood glucose levels increase triglyceride levels, as do being overweight and consuming alcohol, simple sugars, and fat. High-fiber foods, exercise, and weight loss can bring high triglyceride levels down to a safe level—no greater than 150 mg/dL for people with diabetes.

After the Diagnosis

Once diabetes has been diagnosed, you will probably have many questions and concerns. You are not alone: this is the time to gather together your health-care management team. These professionals will answer your questions, help you monitor your disease, and provide medical and emotional support for you. Your primary-care physician or his staff can help you create this network. In addition to your primary-care physician, other members of your health-care management team can include the individuals listed below and on page 40. If possible, find a facility that houses most or all of these professionals, as having a central location will make supervision of your care easier and more satisfying for you.

Health-Care Management Team Approach

For optimum care, a suggested appointment schedule is included in the following information. Naturally, if you are experiencing any problems or have questions between scheduled visits, you need to see the appropriate professional as needed. Based on results of the DCCT, many experts are now recommending you visit your primary-care physician every six months.

In addition to your primary-care physician, two other physicians on your management team may include the following:

• *Diabetologist:* A physician who specializes in diabetes care. Twice-yearly visits are suggested for individuals not taking insulin; the American Diabetes Association recommends a visit every three months for those taking insulin.

• *Endocrinologist:* In the absence of a diabetologist, you may consult with an endocrinologist, who is usually very knowledgeable about diabetes but also specializes in other diseases that involve hormones.

Among your primary-care physician, diabetologist, and/ or endocrinologist, you can expect the following tests and evaluations to be done: a complete physical examination, including eyes and feet; test of blood glucose and glycosylated hemoglobin levels (see "Blood Glucose Testing," pp. 46–49); a urine analysis; measurement of cholesterol and triglycerides; test of kidney function; a test of your glucose monitor against lab results to be sure your monitor is accurate; and a review of your treatment program.

Other members of your team who focus on more individual needs include:

• *Registered Dietitian (R.D.):* This professional can help determine your nutritional needs and work with you to develop a meal plan based on your lifestyle and medical needs. Often this individual is also a certified diabetes educator. Visit at least once a year to review or revise your eating plan or whenever you make a change in your treatment program. If newly diagnosed, you may need to consult your dietitian more often.

• *Diabetes Nurse Educator:* This professional is usually responsible for teaching about insulin therapy, how to self-inject, and how to use oral hypoglycemic pills. A diabetes nurse educator should be someone with whom you have a rapport so you can ask questions easily and without fear. Visit or call once a year, whenever you make a change in your treatment program, or you have questions.

• *Exercise Physiologist:* An exercise physiologist works with you to determine your fitness level, create an exercise program, and make adjustments based on your needs. Visit at least once a year.

• *Ophthalmologist:* A thorough eye examination is recommended once a year to monitor possible development of cataracts, glaucoma, or nerve damage.

• *Podiatrist (Foot Doctor):* If you do daily foot care, a once-yearly visit to your podiatrist is recommended. If routine foot care is a problem for you, two to four times a year may be required.

• *Mental Health Professional:* An individual who is trained to deal with the stresses associated with a chronic disease such as diabetes can be a tremendous help and comfort to you. You may find you need to consult this individual more often soon after diagnosis is made and whenever diabetes disrupts your lifestyle.

Natural Medicine Providers: Whom Should You Call?

After you have been diagnosed with diabetes and have met with your physician and possibly other members of your management team, you may be ready to explore some natural medicine techniques to help you control and manage your diabetes. How do you find natural medicine practitioners? What can they do for you? Appendix A offers a listing of professional organizations that offer referrals and information on natural medicine organizations and practitioners. You also can check the yellow pages of your local telephone directory under individual specialties, such as hypnosis and massage. Other good sources for referrals may be family, friends, and co-workers.

We have divided the natural medicine providers into categories as we did in the Introduction to this book. Who should you call for help with:

• *Nutrition, Nutritional Supplementation, and Herbal Medicine.* Professionals in this category include nutritionists, naturopaths, and herbalists. Naturopaths take a holistic view of diabetes and can provide nutritional advice, exercise programs, and herbal remedies, while nutritionists are more likely to concentrate solely on food and nutrition. Both can consult on weight problems and recommend vitamin supplement regimens. Naturopaths are the only licensed primary health-care practitioners who receive comprehensive training in therapeutic diets and preventive nutrition. They also receive comprehensive training in behavior-oriented counseling. Naturopaths can study at one of the three naturopathic medical schools in the United States, where they complete a four-year doctoral program that leads to the Doctor of Naturopathic Medicine (N.D.) degree.

Nutritionists can have one or more degrees (B.S., M.S., Ph.D.) in nutrition from a college or university, where they can take nutrition, chemistry, microbiology, and anatomy classes. Unfortunately, there are some self-styled nutritionists who received their diplomas from mail-order colleges. Check credentials and get referrals (see Appendix A).

Herbalists consult on the use of plants and their healing qualities. Herbal medicine is not a licensed profession in the United States, and most herbalists are self-taught or train with knowledgeable individuals in the field. Appendix A has several excellent organizations you can contact for information.

• *Movement Therapy.* Before you start any kind of exercise or movement therapy program, consult with your exercise physiologist or your physician. Their role is to help you develop a plan that will make management of your diabetes as easy and stress free as possible. After you get your physician's approval and guidelines, it's up to you to follow through. Refer to the books listed in the Suggested Reading List for additional help.

• *Oxygen Therapy.* This therapeutic approach is alternately considered a natural therapy by those who view oxygen as a natural agent and as a conventional "drug" therapy by those who consider oxygen a drug. We treat it as the former. Its primary application in people with diabetes is for those with poor wound healing. Oxygen therapy can be accessed through more than 260 centers around the country (see Appendix A).

• *Bioenergy Therapy.* This is a very broad category and in this book includes individuals who practice acupressure/

shiatsu, acupuncture, biomagnetic touch healing, homeopathy, polarity therapy, reflexology, and tai chi. Professionals who practice bioenergy therapies manipulate or influence the body's energy field in some way, whether it be laying on of hands, application of pressure, ingestion of natural elements that alter the body's vital force, or slow, focused movement. A homeopath, for example, chooses a natural remedy that not only addresses a particular condition, but also considers your personality and emotional state. Thus the very essence of who you are, your energy, is treated, rather than the "condition."

Training of bioenergy therapists is unique to each discipline. All of the natural therapies in this book have professional organizations you can contact for information and referrals to certified, licensed professionals (see Appendix A).

• *Mind/Body Therapies.* These include breathing therapy, hypnosis, massage, meditation, visualization/guided imagery, and yoga. Practitioners of these natural healing techniques can be found in healing and wellness centers or clinics in many cities; or you may contact an independent professional hypnotherapist, massage therapist, yoga practitioner, or other individuals who practice and teach relaxation and stress-reduction methods through one of the organizations listed in Appendix A or your local yellow pages.

There is often much overlap of skills among professionals in the natural healing techniques. For example, yoga practitioners usually teach and practice breathing techniques and meditation; hypnotherapists often use visualization during their sessions; many massage therapists are trained in reflexology; and some homeopaths practice mind/body therapies. Such multidisciplined practitioners can truly broaden your therapeutic experiences. Reap the benefits of their expertise when you can!

This chapter has offered you signs and signals of diabetes as well as individuals who can help you read and interpret them. Management of your diabetes is a team effort, but you lead the way. The ultimate responsibility—and control—is yours. When you are ready, call upon individuals from the natural medicine arena to help you improve the quality and quantity of that control.

CHAPTER THREE

Guidelines for Daily Management of Diabetes

In Chapter 2, you read about all the people who can be part of your diabetes management team. You can fire any of these people and seek out new ones, but you'll always be left with the most important person on the team: you. You live with diabetes every day of your life, and there are certain routines you need to follow and precautions you should be aware of in order to have the best glucose control and most normal life possible. In this chapter we discuss some of the guidelines for everyday self-care, such as monitoring blood sugar levels; creating an exercise routine; dealing with meals away from home; caring for your feet and teeth; choosing tobacco, alcohol, and other drugs; travel tips; handling hypoglycemia; and coping with illness.

Monitoring Your Diabetes

Because your body can no longer regulate your blood glucose without help, you must provide that help daily. To make sure you're on the right track and keeping your blood glucose levels within normal range, you need to "check in" several times a day. Experts recommend monitoring blood glucose levels even if you do not take insulin. Never mind if you feel all right and don't think you need to monitor. Many people don't have symptoms when their glucose is moderately out of control. The trick is to catch fluctuations before they **do** cause symptoms and any more damage to your body.

In fact, the Diabetes Control and Complications Trial (DCCT) concluded that people with diabetes who keep their blood glucose levels as close to normal as possible can reduce their risk of getting diabetic complications by at least 50 percent. Although this extensive investigation studied Type I diabetes only, the experts feel confident that this same approach will be effective in people with Type II diabetes as well.

With all of these things in mind, the American Diabetes Association recommends that, at the very least, you test your blood glucose levels if you have diabetes and you are:

- Taking insulin
- Following an intensive (tight control) insulin program
- Pregnant
- Having a difficult time controlling your blood glucose levels
- Experiencing low blood glucose (hypoglycemia) levels without the usual warning signs
- Experiencing severe low blood glucose levels or ketones caused by high blood glucose levels

Blood Glucose Testing

The most accurate way to test your glucose levels is to use a blood testing device. Two methods are available, and both involve pricking one of your fingers with an instrument called a lancet to obtain a drop of blood for testing.

There are several finger-pricking instruments on the market. Your diabetes educator can help you choose the best one for you.

One of the testing methods involves placing a drop of blood on a test strip that has been chemically treated. The strip turns different colors depending on the amount of sugar in the blood. Once the strip has turned color, you compare the color on the strip with colors on a chart that indicates the amount of glucose in your blood. If you have poor eyesight or are color blind, this method will not work well for you.

A second method involves using a handheld device called a blood glucose meter. After you place a drop of blood on a test strip or a cartridge that comes with the meter, the meter measures the level of blood glucose and displays the reading on a screen. If you use a glucose meter, follow directions carefully in order to get accurate readings. Your diabetes educator can teach you how to use the meter properly.

Here are some precautions to ensure accurate test results.

- Keep your meter clean. A dirty meter can give false readings.
- Keep the meter at room temperature.
- Bring your meter to your doctor's office and do a self-test at the same time your doctor is doing one for the lab. Your meter results should be within 15 percent of your doctor's.
- Make sure your meter is set up for the type of test strips you are using.
- Keep your test strips in a cool, dry place, and check the dates on them. Do not use outdated test strips.

When to Monitor

There is no one best time to monitor glucose levels. Based on the type of diabetes you have, which medications you take and when, and your lifestyle, you and your management team will decide when you need to monitor your glucose levels. If you use insulin, your monitoring schedule will relate to when you take your medication. Individuals with Type I diabetes usually need at least two injections of insulin a day, and their doctor may recommend monitoring four times daily. If you are following intensive diabetes therapy—a treatment plan recommended by the DCCT whereby you monitor your blood glucose levels very closely and constantly make adjustments to insulin intake, exercise, and diet—you will monitor blood glucose four or more times daily.

If you have Type II diabetes and use insulin, your doctor may recommend that you monitor only twice a day. If you have Type II diabetes and do not use insulin, once a day may be sufficient. More frequent checks may be necessary anytime you significantly change your routine. If, for example, you plan to go on an all-day hike with friends or you are switching to a new oral hypoglycemic pill, you may need to monitor more often for a day or so.

Monitoring for Ketones

Sometimes you need to test your urine for ketones (see Chapter 1), especially if you are ill or your blood glucose is higher than 240 mg/dL and you have Type I diabetes. High ketone levels in the urine are much more common in Type I diabetes than in Type II and can cause a medical emergency called ketoacidosis if blood glucose levels are also high (see Chapter 1).

There are several products on the market for monitoring ketones. All are nonprescription, simple to use, and accurate. In one product, you place a drop of urine on a tablet and wait to see if the tablet changes color. In two other products, test strips are dipped into a urine sample and the resultant colors are compared with those on a color chart.

Logging Your Results

Periodically, record your blood glucose and ketone levels in a log or record book for a number of days in a row. Also record your insulin or diabetes pill doses; any significant changes in your exercise program, diet, or stress levels; and any hypoglycemic reactions. See Figure I-2, p. 50, for an example of a log sheet. Feel free to make adjustments that fit your situation. Always include a "Comments" column to mark down anything that may explain why you had a particular response that day. Bring your logbook with you when you visit your health-care team members so they can see where adjustments may need to be made.

Exercise: Make It Enjoyable and Effective

We're not going to tell you all the benefits exercise can offer you in the control of diabetes: you can read about that in Part II (see "Movement Therapy"). Here we want to share some tips on getting started and how to keep it going.

Because exercise is such a critical part of effective diabetes management, it's to your advantage to have a good attitude about it and to approach it with your eyes open. That means a positive attitude will make your exercise sessions enjoyable, and knowing what to expect and what your limitations are can eliminate any stress or hesitation you may feel about exercise. With that in mind, here are some guidelines to help put enjoyment and effectiveness into your movement therapy sessions.

DIABETES MONITORING RECORD

Patient's full name _____

Street _____

City & State _____

Date 19	Glucose Test Results						Insulin								Comments
							Before Breakfast		Before Lunch	Before Supper		Bedtime			
	Before Break-fast	Before Noon Meal	Before Supper	At Bedtime	Other		Reg.	Long/Inter.	Reg.	Reg.	Long/Inter.	Reg.	Long/Inter.		

Key: Reg. = Regular or Clear Insulin
Inter. = Intermediate-acting insulin; NPH or Lente
Long = Long-acting insulin; Ultralente

In "Comments" section above record variations in activity; food consumption, or timing, and hypoglycemic reactions.

General Comments: _____
_____
_____

Fig. I-2

Moving for Enjoyment and Effect

• See your physician before starting an exercise program. The American Diabetes Association recommends that anyone with diabetes who is older than thirty-five years should have a stress test before starting an exercise program (see Chapter 2). Some physicians also recommend a stress test for anyone who has had diabetes for more than ten years.

• Ask questions of your physician or exercise therapist who handles your exercise program. It's important for you to understand the intimate relationship between exercise and diabetes. Knowledge is power!

• Choose activities that you enjoy, or find ways to make them enjoyable. If you used to enjoy swimming as a teenager but now, twenty-five years and thirty pounds later, you don't want to be seen in a swimsuit, find a way to make it comfortable for yourself. Perhaps you can join a water aerobics class for people with a weight problem or find a pool where you can swim during "off" hours.

• Mix it up! Having a variety of activities from which to choose helps prevent boredom, reduces the risk of injury, and can provide you with better overall fitness. You might jog on Monday, take an aerobics class with a friend on Tuesday and Thursday, use a rowing machine on Friday, and walk on Sunday. Or you might switch back and forth between two of your favorite activities every other day.

• Do it with a friend or group. A thirty-minute jog goes by much quicker when you have a buddy to chat with along the way. Or you might join an exercise class or health club.

• Fit your exercise comfortably into your daily schedule. If you are tense or feel "rushed" to "get it over with," you will not get the benefits you need. You may need to adjust your schedule. For example, you may find that taking a brisk forty-minute walk after work—rather than getting in your car and sitting in traffic—not only allows you to unwind at the end of the day, it may also get you home only a few minutes later than when you left the office at quitting time. Other tips include: Take a walk during your lunch break (but don't skip lunch!) or during coffee breaks; walk to do your errands whenever possible; get off the bus a few blocks before your destination and walk the rest of the way; walk inside an indoor mall when the weather is poor.

• Make exercise part of your vacation plans. It's also a great time to start an easy movement-therapy program, such as walking, jogging, or biking, because it will have the air of adventure!

• Establish goals and rewards for yourself. You might set a goal and chart your progress or get friends or co-workers to join you. For example, you and a group of your friends may live in Milwaukee and decide to walk to Orlando, Florida. Calculate the miles to Orlando and make up a chart that lists each person's name and how many miles he or she walks each week. The first person to walk the total number of miles to reach Orlando gets a special reward—perhaps lunch or theater tickets.

• Visualize yourself as a person who feels good, looks good, and has lots of energy. Know that you are doing good things for yourself. Imagery and self-hypnosis can help you here (see "Hypnosis" and "Visualization and Guided Imagery").

Safety First: Movement Therapy Precautions

If you are taking insulin or oral hypoglycemic medication, heed these safety tips when exercising.

• Learn to recognize the signs that your blood glucose levels are falling. See Chapter 1 for a list of signs of hypoglycemia.

• Test your blood glucose before and after exercise to track how your activity is affecting you. Your insulin or oral medication needs may change as you exercise. If you plan on participating in a physical activity for more than one hour, take your blood glucose meter with you to check your levels halfway through your session.

• Carry fast-acting carbohydrate foods with you as a precaution. Raisins and other dried fruit, fruit juice, or hard sugar candy are easy to take.

• Be aware of "hypoglycemic unawareness," a type of hypoglycemia that hits suddenly without any warning symptoms. This is most common among people who have had diabetes for more than ten years. It is believed this occurs because the body no longer releases the adrenaline that causes hypoglycemic warning signals. To avoid these "sneak" attacks, check your blood glucose levels often during and after exercise, always carry glucose tablets, and consult with your physician.

• If you must stop exercising for a while because of illness, injury, or other circumstances, begin gradually when you start exercising again. Sudden shifts in activity level can affect your blood glucose.

• Bring a friend along if you plan to exercise in an isolated area, especially if you are prone to hypoglycemia.

• Always wear a diabetes identification bracelet or necklace or at least carry identification that gives your name, address, phone number, doctor's name and phone number, insulin requirements, and other medications you take.

The Best Time to Exercise

Many physicians believe the best time to exercise is when your blood glucose level is highest. This differs for every person, so you will need to consult with your physician or exercise physiologist to determine what time of the day is best for you. Not everyone can fit the "best" exercise time into his or her schedule, however, so you may need to be flexible. Here are some general guidelines to choosing exercise times.

• To determine when your blood glucose levels are highest, track your levels over a twenty-four-hour period for several days and place them on a chart.

• If you are concerned about controlling your blood glucose levels, it is usually best to exercise about ninety minutes after eating. This helps prevent your blood glucose from rising as high as it normally does after a meal. If you are taking insulin, exercise after eating to protect against developing hypoglycemia.

• If your blood glucose levels are not low in the morning, that may be the best time for you to exercise. Movement therapy in the morning can lower glucose levels for many hours and help you stay alert all day.

• Avoid exercising before you go to bed, because there is a chance your blood glucose level will continue to drop while you sleep, and you won't know it.

Avoiding Food Fights

You already know that good nutrition and planned eating patterns are crucial for effective diabetes management. In Part II under "Nutrition," we look at several nutritional eating plans in depth. Here, we look at some frustrating situations that arise about food that are outside the realm of eating plans, such as eating out and how to read food labels.

Eating Out

Having diabetes doesn't mean you can't ever eat out again. When you first learn you have diabetes, you may be wary about going to a restaurant or a friend's house for dinner. Here are some survival tips to help avoid food phobia!

• Choose restaurants that offer "heart-healthy" items. Many restaurants are putting these items on their menus because the public is demanding them . . . and not just people with diabetes!

• Avoid fast-food restaurants and steak houses. They tend to serve up lots of high-fat, high-cholesterol, high-sodium, low-fiber foods. Even if there are a few items on the menu that are healthy, you may be tempted to "slip."

• If you are part of a group that is going to a restaurant, speak up if you are unfamiliar with their choice. Call ahead and make sure they can accommodate your needs. Restaurant owners want to keep their customers happy.

• Avoid "all-you-can-eat" restaurants. What sounds like a bargain is usually an invitation to overeating. Even innocent salad bars are often laden with cheese, eggs, and high-fat salad dressings that may be hard to resist.

• Ask questions of the wait staff. Ask how certain items are cooked and served. A baked potato or dish of pasta becomes a nightmare if buried under butter and cheese sauces. *Stir fried* sounds safe, but ask if unsaturated oil, such as canola, corn, or olive oil, is used. Ask for sauces and condiments on the side.

• If you don't see an entree that you want, order from the appetizer and salad columns. A bowl of minestrone soup, a dinner salad, and a baked potato is a perfect meal.

• Try to judge portion sizes. The restaurant's portions may be larger than your usual serving. To avoid temptation, judge what your serving size should be and push the extra off to the side of your plate. Now you have a doggie-bag item!

• If you are following the food-exchange eating plan, you may want to carry a pocket-sized food-exchange list with you to help you while you eat away from home.

• If someone who is not familiar with your needs invites you to his or her home for dinner, let the host know before the event that you have some dietary needs. Although it may seem awkward, it is better to make adjustments before the dinner than to be faced with foods you cannot eat.

• Timing is everything. When eating out and you have some say in when the meal will be served, voice your preferences. If the group asks, "What time should we meet for dinner?" choose a time that is near your usual dinner hour. If you have no control—such as a wedding reception—you may need to have a snack and adjust your medication before the event. Make sure you include the calories you eat at the snack as part of your daily intake.

• Be prepared for delays. Even the best-laid plans can go awry. The invitation may say dinner at six but the guest of honor is delayed and by seven-thirty there's still no sign of food. Keep small carbohydrate snacks with you to ward off hypoglycemia and, if on insulin, bring your medication and syringe with you.

• Alcohol is often a part of social events. It is usually best to avoid alcohol altogether (see "Choosing Alcohol, Tobacco, and Other Drugs," pp. 60–65). Substitute with a club soda with a twist, a diet soda, or a nonalcoholic beer. If you wish to include alcohol in your diet, consult with your physician first.

Reading Food Labels

Thanks to new labeling regulations by the Food and Drug Administration (FDA), all U.S. food products must carry a label with "Nutrition Facts." We will briefly explain the items that appear on these labels.

The **serving size** may or may not be the amount you normally eat. You need to decide what your serving size will be, as this figure determines whether you will need to recalculate the remaining items. Under **total fat,** look for monounsaturated fats or polyunsaturated fats. These are the "good" fats and come from vegetable rather than animal sources. Avoid products that contain saturated fats, such as beef fat, lard, butter, palm oil, or coconut oil.

Check the **cholesterol** figure against the recommended amount in your eating plan, which can range from zero to no more than 300 mg/day, depending on the plan. When you come to **sodium** and you want to keep your sodium intake down, select foods that have less than 400 mg for a single serving. **Total carbohydrate** has two figures under it: dietary fiber and sugars. The total carbohydrate figure and the **protein** figure are the important ones to consider when determining the amount of carbohydrate, protein, and fat (total fat) you consume per day.

The ingredients are listed in descending order by weight. If you plan to use the ADA's food exchange eating plan, you will need to calculate which and how many food groups are represented by each food item you choose. There are several excellent books on how to do food exchanges; see the Suggested Reading List. If, however, you use any of the other eating plans explained in Part II under "Nutrition," no additional calculations are necessary.

Interpreting Label Terms

In May 1994, the FDA mandated that the following terms used on food labels would be defined as stated below.

- *Low fat* means no more than 3 grams of fat per serving.
- *Low in saturated fat* means no more than 1 gram of saturated fat per serving or no more than 15 percent of total calories are from saturated fat.
- *Low sodium* means each serving has 140 mg or less of sodium.
- *Light, Lite* means the food has one third fewer calories or 50 percent less fat per serving.
- *Low cholesterol* means no more than 20 mg of cholesterol and 2 grams or less of saturated fat per serving.

• *Percent fat free* can be used only on foods that are low fat or fat free already.

Foot Care

People with diabetes spend more time in the hospital because of foot problems than for any other condition. (See Chapter 1, ''Foot Problems,'' p. 22) This occurs for several reasons, all associated with other complications that can accompany diabetes. These reasons include:

• Less feeling in the feet because of nerve damage (neuropathy). This can make it impossible to feel cuts and other injuries or to detect extremes in temperature.
• Blockage or narrowing of the blood vessels causes poor circulation in the feet.
• Obesity makes it hard to reach down and properly inspect the feet.
• Poorly managed diabetes often leads to a weakened immune system, and thus a higher risk of infection.
• Eye problems can make it difficult to adequately see foot problems.

Below we present you with quick tips that can help you prevent foot problems. Take a few moments each day to care for your feet, and they will take care of you.

• Wash your feet in warm, soapy water daily. Do not soak them, and do not use hot water. Test the temperature of the water with your elbow. Dry your feet thoroughly and carefully.
• While drying your feet, inspect them carefully, especially between the toes. If you can't see the bottoms, place a hand mirror on the floor or against the wall and put your feet near it. Look for cracks, dryness, sores, swelling, and discoloration. Contact your physician if you see any problem areas.

• Once you have inspected your feet, apply a nonperfumed moisturizer cream. Do not, however, put cream between your toes. If your feet perspire, use a mild foot powder or baby powder to absorb the moisture.

• While you're down there, check your toenails. Keep them short and filed. If you have trouble reaching or seeing your toes clearly, ask a partner, friend, or a member of your health team to clip your nails for you. Do not use scissors or clippers, as you may cut yourself and possibly cause an infection. If you see any nail abnormalities such as thickening or discoloration, advise your physician.

• Check your feet for corns, calluses, blisters, and warts. Do NOT attempt to remove these skin problems yourself. Corns and calluses can develop into foot ulcers and so should be seen by a foot doctor. Treat blisters with antiseptic. If a wart is painful or changes shape or size, consult your physician or foot doctor.

• Wear properly fitted shoes and ones that offer adequate protection. Bare feet and sandals are not recommended, as they leave your feet open to injury. Avoid shoes that squeeze your toes or restrict the blood circulation in your feet.

• Wear nonrestrictive socks and stockings to allow good circulation. If your feet sweat, change your socks or stockings several times a day to avoid infection. Cotton and wool socks and stockings are preferred.

• Be aware of extremes in temperature. Do not walk barefoot on sand or a hot pavement, check bath water before stepping in, and be careful in saunas and hot tubs. Wear adequate protection against frostbite in cold weather.

• When treating cuts and scratches on your feet, wash the area with warm water and mild soap. Dry carefully. Homeopathic remedies for cuts include calendula (available as lotion and oil for cuts and scratches) and hypericum (liquid). Consult your physician or homeopath. You also can use mild antiseptics such as Bactine. Never use harsh antiseptics such as iodine, boric acid, Epsom salts, or mercurochrome.

Dental Care

Poor blood glucose control can lead to gum infection and gum disease. Preventive measures to take include the following:

- Brush after each meal. Use a soft toothbrush and fluoride toothpaste with baking soda.
- Floss at least once a day.
- Have a dental examination every six months.
- Go to a dentist who knows how to treat an insulin reaction.
- If you need dental work that requires anesthesia, consult with your physician as well as your dentist.
- Time your dental visits to avoid insulin reactions.
- Go to your appointments prepared to test your blood glucose levels if your visit takes longer than you expected.

Choosing Tobacco, Alcohol, and Other Drugs

Making wise choices about the use of tobacco, alcohol, and prescription, nonprescription, and illegal drugs is everyone's individual responsibility. All of these substances can have a significant effect on diabetes.

Alcohol

Alcohol is a drug that should be used responsibly. Although many people with diabetes can drink alcohol, moderation is the key. Check with your physician before you decide to make alcohol a part of your lifestyle.

A moderate amount of alcohol is considered to be equal to one or two "alcohol equivalents" a day, with each alcohol equivalent being equal to:

- a 12-ounce light beer;
- a mixed drink containing 1.5 ounces of hard liquor (rye, vodka, scotch, gin) mixed with a sugar-free soda. (Regular soda, juices, and mixes have too many calories and carbohydrates.) These drinks should be spread out over two hours or more.

Alcohol can cause many complications for people with diabetes.

- Alcohol can cause very low blood glucose reactions in people who take insulin or diabetes pills. This occurs because while the alcohol is being processed in the liver, the liver stops doing its regular job, which is to release sugar into your bloodstream. You can experience a hyperglycemic reaction up to thirty-six hours after drinking.
- Alcohol can contribute to obesity. Not only is it full of empty calories, alcohol also can stimulate the appetite.
- Speaking of empty calories, you must count the calories you consume from alcohol into your daily eating plan. If you use the food exchange system, you need to choose the appropriate equivalent.
- If you have nephropathy, alcohol can make it worse.
- If you are taking a diabetes pill called Diabinese and you drink alcohol, you may experience headaches and facial flushing. These are temporary, but annoying, symptoms.
- Sweet wines, cordials, and liqueurs are very high in calories and contain high amounts of carbohydrates. They should be avoided.

Tobacco

The recommendation about smoking is simple: don't. Nicotine narrows the blood vessels and increases your risk of blood vessel disease. This is bad for everyone, but people with diabetes are especially susceptible to blood vessel disease and stroke.

If you smoke, get help and quit. It takes commitment and a change in attitude, but it can be the most positive change you make in your life. To help make quitting easier, consider the following suggestions:

• Make a commitment to quit. Do whatever it takes—make a bet with someone or go to a hypnotherapist or a stop-smoking clinic. Ask your management team for help.

• Give away all your ashtrays and throw away all your cigarettes and lighters.

• Stay away from usual smoking places.

• Whenever you get a craving for a cigarette, take a walk, brush your teeth, drink some water, or practice breathing exercises or yoga.

• Avoid caffeine and alcohol.

• Adopt new, healthy habits to replace your smoking. Some people find that taking up a new sport or exercise when they quit smoking helps them get rid of the stress associated with quitting. Brisk walking, jogging, tai chi, and yoga are easy to do. Remember to monitor your blood glucose levels carefully when starting new activities.

Drugs

Many prescription and nonprescription drugs can cause side effects and drug interactions with insulin or any diabetes pills you may be taking. Table I-4 gives a brief overview of the effects of some over-the-counter medications on diabetes and its complications. Always consult with your physician or pharmacist before taking any nonprescription or prescription drug, including aspirin. (See Part III.)

TABLE I-4
EFFECTS OF OVER-THE-COUNTER DRUGS ON DIABETES AND DIABETIC COMPLICATIONS

Type of Drug	Examples	Effects
Aspirin	Anacin, Bufferin, Bayer, Ecotrin, Excedrin	May increase effect of diabetes pills; may worsen kidney function in people with nephropathy
Ibuprofen	Advil, CoAdvil, Motrin, Nuprin, and others	May worsen kidney function in people with nephropathy
Decongestants	Sudafed and others	May raise blood glucose and blood pressure, worsen retinopathy, heart disease
Antihistamines	Chlor-Trimeton and others	May cause dry mouth, confusion, drowsiness, urinary retention, constipation; may worsen glaucoma
Cough medicine	Benylin, Formula 44, Robitussin, Triaminic	Many contain alcohol and/or sugar; may cause drowsiness
Combination	Actifed, Contac, NyQuil, Sudafed Plus, and others	Consult physician or pharmacist

Type of Drug	Examples	Effects
Diet Pills	Dexatrim, Acutrim, Appedrine, and others	May increase blood pressure, worsen retinopathy, cause "jitters"
Sleep Aids	Nytol, Compoz, Unisom	Same as antihistamines

Some drugs can increase blood glucose levels. These include caffeine, which is found in coffee, tea, cola, and some nonprescription and prescription drugs. Check the labels of over-the-counter medications for caffeine content. Other drugs known to raise blood glucose levels include:

- Thiazide diuretics (e.g., Diuril, Dyazide, Esidrix, Maxzide, and others)
- Corticosteroids (e.g., Cortef, Decadron, Deltasone, Medrol, and others)
- Estrogen (e.g., Norinyl, Premarin, and others)
- Phenytoin (Dilantin)
- Calcium channel blockers (e.g., Adalat, Calan, Procardia, and others)
- Cyclosporine (Sandimmune)
- Encainide (Enkaid)

There are also drugs that can decrease blood glucose levels and cause hypoglycemia. Some of these include:

- Beta-blockers (e.g., Inderal, Tenormin, Lopressor, Visken, and others)
- Anabolic steroids (e.g., Durabolin, Deca-Durobolin, Maxibolin, and others)
- Salicylates (e.g., Anacin, Ascriptin, Bayer, Empirin, and others)

- Monoamine oxidase inhibitors (e.g., Marplan, Nardil, Parnate, and others)

Illegal drugs such as heroin, crack, marijuana, and cocaine have devastating effects on the body and can make management of diabetes impossible. Streets drugs can seriously affect your ability to recognize insulin reactions and to remember to follow your diabetes medication schedule or meal plans. If you have a problem with street drugs, allow your management team to guide you to the help you need to quit.

Travel Tips

Having diabetes need not restrict your travel plans, whether you want to go camping, hike in the mountains, drive around the country, cruise the Caribbean, or fly to Europe. Just like anyone else, it is best to plan ahead so you won't have any surprises that upset your trip.

Here are some suggestions to consider when you plan your next trip. We have tried to cover all types of trip circumstances, from short, overnight driving excursions to extended stays in a foreign country.

- When driving, keep a supply of carbohydrates with you. If you begin to feel even mild symptoms of low blood glucose, pull over to the side of the road and eat 15 grams of carbohydrate. You can now buy carbohydrate paste in a tube that simply squeezes into your mouth. Wait until your symptoms go away before driving again.
- Always wear a medical ID bracelet or neck chain that shows you have diabetes and gives an emergency phone number. Also always carry identification in your wallet or purse that gives your name, address, phone number, doc-

tor's name and phone number, and type and dose of insulin and other medications you take.

• If planning an extended trip or one that takes you out of the country, have a medical examination before you go. You may want to get a letter from your doctor that explains your condition and any complications in the event you seek medical help from another physician while you are away. The letter can also explain any medications and syringes you may be carrying in case you are questioned.

• Take extra insulin, syringes, diabetes pills, and other medications with you, as well as the prescriptions for them. Keep a record of the generic names of your medications, as brand names vary from country to country.

• If the insulin you normally take is not available in the area you are visiting, ask your doctor for a prescription for an alternative form. If possible, however, bring along all the insulin you will need from home.

• If you are crossing time zones, work with your physician or nurse educator to make up a medication schedule that takes time differences into account.

• Avoid fatigue. If crossing several time zones, you may get overtired without realizing it. Be sure to get enough rest.

• Have the name of a doctor you can contact in the area you plan to visit. Contact your local or national American Diabetes Association or, for travel in foreign countries, the International Diabetes Center (see Appendix A) for assistance.

• If you are traveling to a foreign country, learn how to say, "I have diabetes," "Please give me sugar or orange juice," and "Please call a doctor" in the appropriate language. Write these phrases down and carry them with you.

• For airline travel, bring your insulin, syringes, diabetes pills, other medications, and snacks in your carry-on luggage.

• Don't forget to exercise while traveling. If driving, stop and take a brief walk every one and one half to two hours. If on a plane or train, walk up and down the aisles to stimulate circulation. During bus trips, use the rest stops as a time for a walk.

• Prevent motion sickness and diarrhea. Ask your management team for recommended motion-sickness medication before you leave. If you're traveling to a foreign country, diarrhea can be a problem. To prevent it, stay away from peeled fruit, leafy vegetables, meats, and dairy products. Drink only bottled water and tea or packaged sodas. Do not drink tap water, even to brush your teeth, or use ice cubes.

• Continue to monitor your blood glucose levels regularly. Traveling can present you with changes in eating and sleeping patterns, unusual foods, different activity levels, and other stresses.

Handling Hypoglycemia

You can prevent or reduce the severity of hypoglycemic episodes by monitoring your blood sugar levels often and becoming familiar with the symptoms of low blood sugar (see Chapter 1) and circumstances in your life that may trigger them. Consult with your physician to determine the blood glucose level that is optimal for you. Your safest blood sugar level depends on your age, medical condition, and ability to recognize hypoglycemic symptoms. People with diabetes often are attuned to when their blood sugar levels are dropping and can reverse the situation by eating or drinking something with sugar in it. One of the things the natural-medicine practices explained in this book do is increase your awareness of your body so you are better able to recognize and manage hypoglycemia.

Hypoglycemia is usually caused by poor timing of meals

or snacks; other causes include exercising more than normal without adjusting your insulin or food intake, dieting, or taking too much insulin. To manage hypoglycemia, consider the following guidelines.

• Be prepared. Always carry a readily available carbohydrate source with you, such as hard sugar candy, glucose tablets, or raisins. Nuts and chocolate are not recommended, as they contain too much fat.

• If you can, test your blood glucose level to make sure it is low. Sometimes other medical conditions can cause symptoms similar to those of hypoglycemia. If you cannot test, go to the next step.

• Treat it immediately. Even if you are having only mild symptoms, putting off treatment may lead to more serious problems.

• Remain calm. Eat your carbohydrate food and wait ten to fifteen minutes for it to take effect. If it does not, eat some more. If there still is no improvement, call your physician.

• If you take insulin and frequently experience hypoglycemia, consult with your management team. You may need to adjust your insulin doses.

In rare cases, people with Type II diabetes may develop a condition called hypoglycemia unawareness, in which they have difficulty recognizing hypoglycemic symptoms. The remedy for this is an injection of glucagon (by another person), which immediately releases glucose into the bloodstream and relieves the symptoms of low blood sugar (see Part III). If the symptoms do not disappear in a few minutes, emergency medical assistance should be sought.

Pregnancy and Diabetes

Advanced techniques in obstetrical care and diabetes management have made pregnancy and childbirth a much safer experience for women with diabetes. However, strict blood glucose control is essential both before and during pregnancy. Women with diabetes are at higher risk than the general population of having children with birth defects. This risk is greatest during the first few months of pregnancy. Therefore, if you know you are pregnant, are planning a pregnancy, or there is a chance you may become pregnant, maintain tight control of your blood glucose levels and consult with your physician.

During pregnancy you need to add an obstetrician who is knowledgeable about diabetes to your management team. Many physicians recommend that women with diabetes who are pregnant monitor their blood glucose levels four to seven times a day. If you are on insulin, your insulin needs will change, and you will work with your management team to make those changes.

Your nutritional needs will also change. During the first few months of pregnancy you may have a decrease in appetite because of nausea. As your appetite improves, you will add extra calories to your meal plan. Pay particular attention to your evening snack to help prevent hypoglycemia while you sleep. Your baby feeds twenty-four hours a day, and some women find they need to have a snack in the middle of the night to prevent hypoglycemia.

A common concern of women with diabetes who are pregnant is whether their baby will have diabetes. If you have Type I diabetes, the chance of your child developing the disease is 2 percent. If the father has diabetes and you do not, the chance is 4 percent. The risk increases significantly if both you and the father have Type I diabetes: 25 to 30 percent. Some experts believe Type I diabetes is linked with the mother's diet. For a view on how to prevent diabetes during pregnancy, see "Gerson Therapy" under Nutrition in Part II.

Another concern is whether pregnancy increases the risk for developing diabetic complications. If you have nerve, eye, or mild kidney disease, you will probably have a healthy pregnancy if you follow all of your management team's advice. If you have retinopathy and become pregnant, it is recommended you be closely monitored by an eye specialist throughout your pregnancy, as the condition can worsen significantly. Pregnancy is not recommended if you have uncontrolled high blood pressure, heart problems, or advanced kidney disease, as these can place both you and your baby at risk of death.

Dealing with Illness and Diabetes

When people who don't have diabetes become ill with a cold or the flu, they usually don't think twice about taking aspirin, cough suppressants, or something to settle their stomach. When you become ill, however, you need to be aware of potential problems. Some over-the-counter medications, for example, contain caffeine, which can increase blood glucose levels and blood pressure. Cold medications with decongestants also can cause blood glucose levels to increase. Large doses of aspirin can increase the effect of oral hypoglycemic drugs. Although some over-the-counter drug labels warn patients with diabetes, hypertension, and other conditions to take the medications only under their doctor's guidance, it is best to consult your physician before taking *any* medication. (Also see "Choosing Tobacco, Alcohol, and Other Drugs," pp. 60–65.)

Generally, if you have a mild, brief illness, follow the guidelines below.

• If you are taking insulin or oral hypoglycemic medication, it is important that you keep taking your medication.

• Monitor your blood glucose and test your urine for ketones at least four times a day. Infection, fever, dehydration, nausea, and other symptoms of cold or flu can cause your body to release stress hormones, which in turn increases your blood glucose levels.

• If your illness prevents you from eating your regular foods, substitute liquids or soft foods that are high in carbohydrates (for example, whole grain toast or bagel, cooked cereal, orange juice, broth-based soups, soy milk, saltine crackers, yogurt).

• If nausea makes eating or taking oral diabetes drugs a problem, a doctor should be consulted. Not eating can increase the risk of low blood glucose, while stopping oral medications or insulin during illness can lead to very high blood glucose. A doctor may prescribe insulin temporarily for someone with diabetes who can't take medicine by mouth.

• To prevent blood glucose levels from dropping quickly, eat frequent, small meals: about fifty grams of carbohydrates every three to four hours.

• To prevent dehydration, drink at least eight ounces of calorie-free liquid every hour—water, diet soda, or tea. If you are vomiting or are nauseated, take several small sips of liquid every fifteen to thirty minutes and contact your physician.

If any of the following situations occur, call your physician or other health-care team member:

• You are unable to eat regular food for more than one day.
• You can't keep liquids or carbohydrates down for more than eight hours.

- You have diarrhea or are vomiting.
- Your breathing is rapid, you are drowsy, or you lose consciousness.

Another concern when you are ill is the use of nonprescription drugs. If you have diabetes and you get a cold or the flu and reach for nonprescription medications, you need to consider the sugar content of these drugs. Diabetes is harder to handle when you are sick, and the amount of sugar in over-the-counter medications, although small, may be enough to cause a reaction. That's why it's best to choose sugar-free varieties when possible (see Table I-5). Read the label anytime you buy an over-the-counter product, even if it is the same brand you bought last time. Manufacturers occasionally change their formulations. Avoid any drug that contains sucrose, glucose, sorbitol, mannitol, fructose, dextrose, or alcohol.

TABLE I-5
OVER-THE-COUNTER MEDICATIONS
FOR PEOPLE WITH DIABETES

Cough Medicines: Those that contain little or no alcohol and are sugar free include the following: Cerose-DM liquid, Colrex cough syrup, Colrex expectorant syrup, Contact Jr. liquid, Hytuss tablets, Naldecon-DX, Scot-Tussin syrup, Tolu-Sed DM liquid

Decongestants: Dimetane decongestant elixir, Dimetapp elixir, Novahistine elixir, Sinutab maximum strength nighttime liquid, Afrin nasal spray, Neo-Synephrine nose drops

Pain and Fever Medications: Datril, Panadol, Tylenol, generic acetaminophen, Nuprin, generic ibuprofen, Children's Panadol, Dolanex elixir

CHAPTER FOUR

The Mind/Body Connection

You are scheduled to give a speech in front of a hundred people. As you wait on the sidelines to go onto the stage, your hands sweat, your heart rate and breathing rate increase, your blood pressure rises, and your blood glucose level begins to climb. For a person without diabetes, the extra sugar pumped into the bloodstream is used by the cells as extra fuel. But if you have diabetes, hypoglycemia may be on the horizon. For years, doctors and researchers have noted that the blood glucose levels of people with diabetes rise during times of stress. They also have known that high levels of stress hormones, such as adrenaline, can cause blood glucose levels to increase. Although stress does not cause diabetes, it may trigger it in people who are genetically susceptible to diabetes. If you already have diabetes, stress can aggravate it. Thus how well you manage stress can have a significant impact on your ability to control your diabetes.

This chapter explores the role of the mind in the perception, control, and reduction of stress in the management of diabetes. The concept of the mind/body connection—the intricate relationship of cause-and-effect between what you think and feel and how your body responds physiologically—is approached by answering several basic questions: What is stress? What is mind/body medicine? What part do stress and emotions play in the control and management of diabetes? How can I make the mind/body connection work for me? Which natural therapies can help me make that connection?

What Is Stress?

You're stuck in a traffic jam and you haven't moved ten feet in as many minutes. Your car isn't overheating yet, but you are. You feel trapped and angry, and the muscles in your neck and shoulder are beginning to hurt. You know you shouldn't let the situation bother you, but you already feel a tension headache coming on and you're beginning to feel light-headed.

In the car next to you is an individual about your age. He or she is singing along with the song on the radio and tapping out a beat on the steering wheel. After a while this person picks up a newspaper from the front seat, folds it carefully, and begins to read.

The same scenario, two different responses to stress. Situations that trigger negative stress responses in one person may elicit little or no negative response from another. Thus the definition of **stress** is not what happens to *you*—the stressors, or outside forces that have the potential to cause stress symptoms—but *how you react to what happens*.

How People with Diabetes Respond to Stress

There are dozens of ways we respond to stress (see Table I-6, p. 77). In addition, research studies show that how we deal with any given stressful situation is determined by many psychological, social, and physical factors, such as our mood at the time the stressor occurs, repressed feelings, age, sex, race, heredity, amount of social support from family and friends, state of our health, and more. One way the body responds to stress is to increase the level of blood glucose. In a person with diabetes, stress may increase the need for insulin or oral hypoglycemic medication in order to lower those raised blood glucose levels. Emotional and psychological stress can be reduced using various stress-management techniques. Physical stress, such as a cold, the flu, or a fracture, may require medical intervention.

How you react to stress is determined largely by a part of the nervous system called the **autonomic nervous system.** This system has two branches, the **sympathetic nervous system** and the **parasympathetic nervous system.** It's the parasympathetic system that helps the body relax by lowering heart rate and blood pressure and relieving muscle tension. This positive response was under investigation by Herbert Benson, M.D., of Harvard Medical School in 1968, when he and his colleagues conducted studies of the effects of meditation on breathing rate, brain-wave patterns, and other physical factors. They discovered that the mind can affect physical functions and set into motion its own stress-reduction mechanisms, and called this reaction the **relaxation response.** Some ways to induce this response for help in dealing with diabetes include meditation, visualization, breathing therapy, yoga, and tai chi, among others. These natural approaches can complement your traditional diabetes management program and are discussed in Part II of this book.

Diabetes Has Unique Stressors

Although stress is part of everyone's life, people with diabetes have some unique stressors. Here are a few that you and other people with diabetes confront daily.

• Diabetes doesn't go away—it is a chronic condition. That doesn't mean you have to *like* it. If you're like nearly everyone who has been diagnosed with diabetes, you have gone through many different emotions about it. Shock and confusion are usually followed by denial—it couldn't happen to you. Fear and anxiety are common reactions, and ones that your management team can help you eliminate. Once you accept your condition, you can learn to control it and minimize any complications so you can get on with your life. There will still be days when you get angry about having diabetes, but those days can be better once you know of ways to manage the disease.

• Diabetes is invisible. As long as you keep your blood glucose level within normal range, no one will know you have diabetes. But *you* know you have to watch what you eat, sometimes restrict your activities, monitor your glucose levels, and take medication. The feeling of appearing to be like everyone else and yet being different can be stressful. When you're out with friends or co-workers, you know you need to keep track of what you eat and when and how active you are. Be patient and allow yourself time to adapt to your new lifestyle.

• The frustration of "why me?" Frustration can make you feel overwhelmed by the disease and having to deal with it. When you are frustrated, you don't feel like doing the things you need to do. You can lose your motivation to stay on target. When we asked people with diabetes what frustrated them the most, they said, "worrying about having an insulin reaction," "having to exercise regularly," "feeling different from other people," and "knowing diabetes will never go away." Much of this frustration can be reduced or eliminated by integrating natural healing practices into your lifestyle. Because natural therapies work with your body and your vital energy instead of introducing something foreign to it, you can have a better sense of yourself and better control of your condition.

• Diabetes is unpredictable. Something as simple as a cold or a cross-country flight can throw off your blood glucose level. If you learn as much as you can about your condition and many different, natural ways to deal with the stresses in your life, you can greatly reduce or eliminate the unpredictability of diabetes.

One area of important research has been in the effect of stress on the immune system. This branch of study, called psychoneuroimmunology (*psycho* for mind, *neuro* for the neuroendocrine system—the hormone and nervous systems—and *immunology* for the immune system) indicates that stress hormones have a role in many diseases, including diabetes, and some of the conditions associated with it, such as hypertension and heart disease. Beyond the basic preventive approaches to dealing with stress, such as good nutrition, adequate sleep, and enough exercise, stress-reduction therapies like those offered in this book are recommended, as is sharing your thoughts and feelings with a therapist or a support network.

TABLE I-6
SYMPTOMS OF STRESS

Are you experiencing some of these stress symptoms? If so, they may be affecting your blood glucose levels.

Physical: stiff or tense muscles, sweating, headache, grinding teeth, feeling faint, difficulty in swallowing or feeling like you are choking, stomach pain, nausea, vomiting, loose bowels, constipation, fatigue, tremors or shakiness, weight gain or loss, awareness of heartbeat, loss of interest in sex, frequent and urgent urination.

Emotional and Cognitive: feeling tense, irritable, restless, worried, depressed; unable to relax; poor concentration, problems with memory, anxious thoughts

Behavioral: crying, difficulty completing tasks, sleep problems, tremors, fidgeting, clenching fists, strained or pinched face, changes in eating, drinking, or smoking habits

What Is Mind/Body Medicine?

Hippocrates, the Father of Medicine, believed health is a state of harmony that exists among the mind, body, spirit, and the external environment. He said, "The natural healing force within each one of us is the greatest force in getting well"; thus we all possess the power to heal ourselves, to some degree, once we integrate and balance the mind, body, and spirit with our surroundings. Natural therapies support this concept because they are based on and work with the mind/body connection.

The growing realization and evidence that mind/body techniques such as meditation, yoga, visualization, hypnosis, and relaxation therapies have a significant effect on disease has blossomed into what is commonly called **mind/body medicine.** This new approach in medical science has several basic concepts: that the mind has a central effect on physical health; that the best way to heal is to treat the whole person; that people should take an active part in their own health care; and that by exercising psychological control, people can prevent or reduce the effects of disease.

Mind/body medicine plays a significant role in diabetes, as stress is a major factor to consider in the management and control of the disease. The success of stress-reduction therapies in diabetes varies among individuals. Your response will depend on the state of your diabetes and other medical conditions, and how conscientious you are about doing the therapy.

The Role of Stress and Emotions in Diabetes

Deepak Chopra, M.D., author of *Perfect Health, Ageless Body, Timeless Mind,* and other books, explains the link between mind/emotion and body: "Mind and body are inseparably one. . . . A basic emotion such as fear can be described as an abstract feeling or as a tangible molecule of the hormone adrenaline. Without the feeling there is no hormone; without the hormone there is no feeling."

The question as to how these feelings and thoughts can impact the development and course of diabetes became the focus of the work of Richard S. Surwit, Ph.D., and Mark Feingloss, M.D., who created the Duke Neurobehavioral Diabetes Program in 1989. Their research and that of other investigators continues today and indicates that healthy management of emotions and attitudes is a key factor in keeping blood glucose levels under control. Healthy management includes use of natural therapies to complement and often reduce your dependence on medical treatment.

Stress can cause fluctuations in blood glucose levels either indirectly or directly. For example, during times of stress, some diabetics don't follow their normal eating plans or they forget to exercise, have trouble sleeping, or skip their medication. Any of these behaviors can cause an increase in blood glucose levels. A more direct cause occurs when, during high-stress situations, the adrenal glands release a large amount of stress hormones such as adrenaline and cortisol into the bloodstream. In people without diabetes, this added sugar is used by the cells as extra fuel. In diabetics, however, it accumulates in the blood and can cause symptoms of hyperglycemia, such as dry mouth, a need to urinate, pain or tingling in the arms or legs, and a sweet or odd taste in the mouth.

Stress has a somewhat different effect on people with Type I than on those with Type II diabetes. In people with Type I diabetes, stress can cause glucose levels to rise in some individuals and fall in others. In those with Type II diabetes, mental stress generally raises blood glucose levels. Physical stress from illness or injury raises blood glucose levels in both types of diabetes.

Management of stress not only helps maintain daily well-being but also helps minimize the complications associated with diabetes, especially heart disease and hypertension. Stress management is also important in preventing depression. Many people with Type II diabetes experience depression. Although depression does not necessarily cause diabetes, it can increase the risk of complications and have a negative impact on overall well-being. People who are seriously depressed have hormonal changes similar to those caused by stress. The result is an increase in the amount of glucose in the blood, which aggravates diabetes.

Depression is common among people with diabetes, especially soon after diagnosis is made or when the disease takes a turn for the worse. A good example is what happens when people with Type II diabetes who have not needed insulin discover they now need it to maintain blood glucose control. Many of these individuals have immediate, but unexpressed, apprehension about this turn of events. They may fear the disease is getting much worse, or that they will develop Type I diabetes. Some will deny anything has changed and insist they feel fine. They may be afraid family or friends may reject them or that taking insulin will change their lives dramatically. Some have a fear of needles.

This psychological resistance to taking insulin has been given a name—PIR, or psychological insulin resistance. PIR is a relatively new name for a distinct condition that affects many people with Type II diabetes who are told to add insulin to their management program. Those who change their attitude about themselves and diabetes through a better understanding of the mind/body connection and commit to make natural stress management techniques a part of their care program can eliminate PIR.

Making the Mind/Body Connection Work for You

Dr. Bernie Siegel believes that "intuitively and instinctively, the unconscious knows what is needed. Our job as individuals confronting disease is to set it free to do its best for us by giving it 'live' messages." "Live" messages can come in several forms. They may be affirmations: "I deserve to feel joy"; "I accept my condition"; "I am a whole and beautiful person with diabetes." Live messages also means loving yourself enough to seek help, follow your diet and exercise program, and try new therapies. If you refuse help or are lax about your diet, you send your body negative messages.

Diabetes is a chronic disease. The last thing your body needs is chronic negative messages. While Dr. Siegel is a strong advocate of using mind/body healing practices such as hypnosis, visualization, meditation, and relaxation techniques in people with chronic disease, "Perhaps more powerful . . . to alter the inner environment of your body are feelings of hope and love."[1] Some people with diabetes develop a fatalistic attitude toward their condition. Naturopath Emily Kane writes that in some people with Type I diabetes, their parents communicated certain powerful messages to them as children, such as: "You're special, but flawed"; "Don't get angry or upset"; "Be independent and don't ever ask for help"; and "You will die young."

1. Bernie S. Siegel, M.D., *Peace, Love & Healing*, p. 115.

Such negative messages leave little room for hope, unless you refuse to listen to this chatter and believe in the power of your own mind and body to improve your life. You may not cure your diabetes, but you can live your life to the fullest. When you love yourself, you will go that one extra step and try yoga or massage or herbal remedies to help control your diabetes and improve your overall health and well-being. The pages that follow can help you do just that.

Natural Therapies and the Mind/Body Connection

An inherent component of natural therapies is their ability to allow people to become more aware of the intimate connection between their mind and body. Any one of the natural therapies discussed in this book, as well as dozens of others that are useful in treating other conditions, can awaken that link and allow you more control over your diabetes.

Perhaps the most popular way natural therapies are used is in stress reduction and management. When stress causes fluctuations in blood sugar and hormone levels, management of diabetes can be difficult. You can use the natural stress reduction therapies discussed in this book, such as meditation, visualization/imagery, biofeedback, and yoga, in two ways: practice them when you get signals from your body that stress is having an impact, such as headache, muscle tension, or signs of hyperglycemia; or, preferably, use them daily to help prevent stress and promote overall well-being. Many people find that beginning each day with ten or fifteen minutes of meditation or visualization, for example, places them in a more relaxed frame of mind. Whether they visualize healing energy racing through their body or lying on a tropical beach; whether they empty their mind and concentrate only on their breath or progressively relax every muscle in their body, they are using their mind to connect with their body. Because they can better cope with daily stresses, they have better control over their blood glucose levels and feel more confident.

Researchers like Dr. Richard S. Surwit have conducted studies in which individuals with Type II diabetes underwent various stress reduction therapies. The results were variable: some people experienced significant control of their diabetes while others got little or no benefit. Generally, people with Type II diabetes who have a high level of stress in their lives show more improvement than those with little stress. Thus far, the few studies of individuals with Type I diabetes and stress reduction techniques have shown little or no increase in blood glucose control. However, stress reduction practices are useful in lowering high blood pressure, a significant problem in many people with diabetes.

We hope this chapter has given you a new perspective on the mind/body connection. Some of the most effective and easy ways to make that connection work for you are explained in Part II. If you want to explore others that are beyond the pages of this book, refer to the Bibliography and Suggested Reading for more ideas.

CAN STRESS REDUCTION HELP CONTROL YOUR DIABETES?

For some individuals with diabetes, relaxation techniques can have beneficial results. The following self-test can help you and your doctor determine if such a course of action might be in your best interests. To ensure success of this assessment, you must not deviate from your medication, diet, and exercise program, and you must know how to properly use a home glucose monitor. The test should be taken over a two-week period.

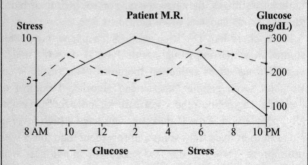

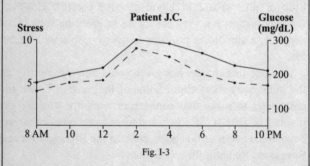

Fig. I-3

You will need to prepare daily charts on graph paper (see Figure I-3). The left vertical axis is your stress level: 1 = no stress and 10 = extreme stress. The right vertical axis is glucose level in mg/dL. Mark the horizontal axis for the intervals at which you check your blood glucose levels; the sample is marked in two-hour intervals. Every time you prepare to test your blood glucose level, first note your stress level and plot it on the graph. Then enter your blood glucose level. Do this throughout each day. Use a different color to draw the lines for the two variables. After two weeks, you should see a pattern. Using a typical day as an example, stress appears to have an impact on blood glucose levels in Patient J.C.: stress and glucose levels rise and fall together. Blood glucose levels in Patient M.R., however, do not seem to be closely tied with stress. Therefore, stress reduction techniques may help patient J.C. but probably will have little or no impact on Patient M.R.

Once you start a stress-reduction program, chart your stress and blood glucose levels again. Any reduction in stress levels hopefully will be accompanied by a reduction in blood glucose. If this is the case, the above plotting exercise can help determine whether relaxation techniques affect your blood glucose levels.

PART TWO

NATURAL HEALING OF DIABETES

Welcome to the "action" part of this book, where we explain some natural ways to manage diabetes, its complications, and factors that affect both, such as stress, nutrition, and exercise. These natural approaches also can be used to prevent or reduce the severity of diabetic complications. There are other natural therapies and methods beyond this book that you can explore; the examples given here introduce you to the scope and diversity of the possibilities in the world of natural healing.

Management of diabetes boils down to a simple equation:

$$\text{Diet} + \text{Exercise} + \text{Stress Management} =$$
$$\text{(hopefully) near normal blood glucose levels}$$

The natural therapies in this section offer you options you may not have considered before in each of the three categories to the left of the equal sign. They are meant to *complement* and augment your current medical treatment for diabetes. None of them will cure diabetes, nor will they replace your current diabetes program. These treatments are *holistic,* which means they consider the whole body in the healing process. When you take care of the whole body, you are much more likely to stay healthy and fit and thus have better control of your blood glucose levels.

As you explore these therapies, keep your mind open to the options. You can always stop doing something that does not appeal to you or help you. Use of any of the natural therapies in this book may, and often will, change your medication requirements. When you decide to include any of these natural approaches as part of your diabetes management program, we strongly recommend that you *first seek out a physician who is knowledgeable about natural healing methods and who is willing to work with you and guide you with your choices.* When working with natural health practitioners, such as homeopaths or naturopaths, keep them informed of your medication status and the level of control you are able to maintain. Together with the guidance of all your health professionals, you can control your diabetes safely and naturally.

Acupressure

Acupressure is an ancient Eastern technique in which the fingers or palms, and occasionally knees or elbows, are used to apply pressure to specific points on the body in order to open up blockages and restore the flow of energy that circulates throughout the body. This energy is often referred to as the "vital force"; in Ayurvedic, it is *prana;* in yogic, *kundalini;* in Taoist, *chi,* pronounced "key." Regardless of the name you attach to it, when you are under stress and have muscle tension, you have an injury, or you are experiencing problems related to poor organ functioning, your vital force can become blocked at the sites of the disorder. When the energy is released, the benefits can include relief from muscle tension, improved organ functioning, better blood circulation, and increased vitality.

The healing traditions of China, India, and Japan are based on a particular understanding of how vital energy moves through the body. According to their teachings, the vital force moves along twelve pathways called *meridians.* Each meridian is associated with a different body system, yet all the systems are interconnected and affect one another. At specific locations along the meridians there are branches that extend both up to the skin's surface and inward toward the organs. The sites at which these branches reach the skin's surface are called acupressure or **trigger points.** Each of these points, of which there are more than 360 on the body, provides an access point to the body's internal energy system. The branches that extend inward keep dividing into smaller and smaller channels that connect to the cells. Thus each of your cells can receive the benefits of released energy from acupressure treatments.

Trigger points are used for treatment by practitioners of acupressure as well as several other, similar therapies, the most popular of which is **shiatsu.** The difference between acupressure and shiatsu is in technique. For example, acupressure therapists and shiatsu practitioners vary in how hard and how long they apply pressure to points and whether they use one hand or two. Some acupressure therapists use their palms, feet, elbows, and even their knees during treatment. Generally, however, the procedures among similar therapies are the same. (See the Bibliography and Suggested Reading for books that describe these and other acupressure techniques.)

THE MERIDIANS AND CORRESPONDING ORGANS

In Figures II-1, II-1a, and II-1b, page 96, the abbreviations *CV, GV,* and so on refer to the meridians through which the vital energy flows and name the acupressure/acupuncture points and their corresponding organs. Acupressure therapists and acupuncturists use these abbreviations when referring to the pressure points.

Lu	Lung	LI	Large Intestine
SP	Spleen	St	Stomach
H	Heart	SI	Small Intestine
K	Kidney	B	Bladder
TW	Triple Warmer	P	Pericardium
LV	Liver	GB	Gall Bladder
CV	Conception Vessel	GV	Governing Vessel

The Conception and Governing vessels run alongside the spinal cord and store energy. Treating the points along these two meridians strengthens and calms the body and also increases the results obtained from stimulation of other points along other meridians.

How Does Acupressure Work?

As your vital force surges through your body, the flow can become blocked because of muscle tension or stress. This includes physical stress (like that associated with a chronic disease such as diabetes, as well as overexercise, injury, or surgery) and mental stress. When you or an acupressure therapist apply pressure to specified trigger points, barriers can be broken down and those points can reconnect with your body's vital force. As these points reconnect, your vital force becomes more balanced and moves toward restoration of optimum energy flow throughout your body.

For individuals with diabetes, acupressure can work on several levels. It can improve blood circulation, stimulate proper functioning of the internal organs, including the pancreas; and help rid the body of toxins. On another level, it can increase your awareness of your body and any signals it gives you about stress levels and other imbalances, such as symptoms of hypoglycemia or hypertension. When your awareness is enhanced, you can act immediately when you sense shifts in body function and ward off negative events.

A Word of Caution

Acupressure increases blood flow and should be avoided if you have any of the following medical conditions. Before treatment begins, tell your acupressure practitioner about any medications you are taking. Properly trained acupressure therapists (see Appendix A for how to find an acupressure practitioner) are aware of the conditions under which acupressure should not be performed.

- Presence of fever or a contagious disease.
- Risk of hemorrhage or thrombosis.
- Osteoporosis.
- Recent tissue damage, bone fractures, or inflammation. Avoid acupressure in the affected areas.
- Pregnancy. Some pressure points on the leg may increase the chance of miscarriage.
- Epilepsy or high blood pressure.

Acupressure for Diabetes

The most beneficial and enjoyable acupressure treatment is a balanced, full-body session. It is usually done in five steps: (1) the shoulders, head, and neck; (2) the back; (3)

the arms and hands; (4) the feet and legs; and (5) the face and front of the body. Each step has specific benefits to people with diabetes. Step 1 energizes the entire body and helps clear up any intestinal problems. Step 2 stimulates all of the major organs. Step 3 is important because it includes working the six meridians that run along the arm, including the heart governor (responsible for blood circulation), triple heater (responsible for caloric energy), and heart meridians. Step 4 includes the kidney, liver, and stomach meridians, while Step 5 continues work on these three meridians and also includes the spleen and gallbladder meridians. To this basic routine can be added specific trigger points to stimulate functioning of the pancreas, liver, adrenal glands, and stomach, which is especially beneficial to people with diabetes. We explain how to treat these specific trigger points on pages 95–96.

A full-body session is best done by a professional acupressure therapist or a spouse or friend who has learned the techniques. The basics can be learned in several hours from a licensed professional or from well-prepared books (see *Basic Shiatsu* by Michio Kushi and others in the Bibliography and Suggested Readings). You also can treat yourself with acupressure: you can probably manage much of a full-body session alone as well as specific points for diabetes once you learn which trigger points you need to work. Before you attempt self-treatment, however, we suggest you have several sessions with a trained, licensed professional and to experience a full-body acupressure session. In this way you can learn firsthand which points to treat, how much pressure to apply, and how a treatment feels. You also might consider taking an introductory course in acupressure.

Here we present trigger points to treat diabetes and some of its associated complications and symptoms.

Specific Trigger Points

Refer to Figure II-1 to find the points discussed below. Using your thumb or index finger, apply light and then increasingly more pressure to each point. Hold the pressure for at least ten seconds and then massage the point by slowly rotating your thumb or finger in a tight circular motion. One to several minutes of firm pressure will help release the blocked energy. You can do these points while sitting comfortably in a chair or lying on a comfortable, firm surface.

• Apply pressure and massage to the points along the spleen meridian, which runs along the inside of the leg (Figure II-1a). Point SP 10 is especially good for stimulating the pancreas and spleen.

• Also along the spleen meridian, locate point SP 6, where the liver, spleen, and kidney meridians intersect. This point is located inside the leg about four finger-widths up from the ankle. DO NOT press this point if you are pregnant.

• Place your thumbs underneath your rib cage. As you exhale, gently press inward and upward on the points shown in Figure II-1b, beginning at CV 14 and the moving to LV 14, GB 24, and LV 13. This is a "mirror image" area, meaning the same points appear on each side of the body. Treat both sides simultaneously. This sequence stimulates the liver, pancreas, spleen, and stomach. Repeat the sequence several times.

• On the bottom of your feet, locate point KD 1, which is in the center of the pads below your toes and directly below the toe next to the big toe. This is where the kidney meridian begins its journey up the inside of the leg. To send energy to your kidneys, massage this point in a counterclockwise direction.

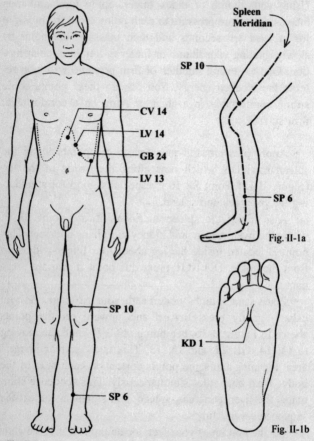

Fig. II-1

Spleen Meridian

SP 10

SP 6

Fig. II-1a

KD 1

Fig. II-1b

CV 14

LV 14

GB 24

LV 13

SP 10

SP 6

As you press and massage all these points, the feeling should be somewhere between pleasure and pain, or a "good hurt." When a blockage is finally released, you will feel a slight pulsing coming from the point. If you don't feel the pulse the first few times you try acupressure, don't be discouraged. It takes time and practice to become sensitive to your body. Acupressure stimulates the body's natural tendency to heal. This process takes time.

For the best results from acupressure, include it as part of your overall diabetes management program, along with other natural therapies. Some people find that using meditation or visualization along with acupressure treatments, for example, enriches their experience.

What to Expect from an Acupressure Therapist

If you need help in finding an acupressure or shiatsu therapist, consult Appendix A. Your treatment will be easiest for the practitioner if you wear comfortable, loose-fitting clothing. The therapist will ask you about your personal and medical history and your pulse will be checked. Tell the practitioner the status of your diabetes, including medications you are taking, how well your glucose levels are controlled, and any complications you may have.

Now it's time for your treatment. Acupressure sessions generally last about one hour. During that time you will be lying on a padded massage or treatment table or on a futon. You may be asked to shift position several times during your session, but it will always be with your comfort in mind. The therapist will press along meridian lines in search of spots where your life energy is blocked. Acupressure therapists believe that soreness around an acupressure point indicates a place where energy flow is blocked. Once a blockage is found, the therapist will press on the point for several seconds or up to two minutes, depending on the practitioner's particular style and beliefs. Individual therapists also differ in how much pressure they apply, whether it be light, deep, or somewhere in between. Many people describe the sensation they feel during treatment as "a good hurt." One or more applications of pressure usually release that hurt and allow your energy to flow freely again.

Acupressure therapists often emphasize that a healthy eating plan that is free of most or all animal products and food additives is most conducive to healing (see "Nutrition"). A healthy diet allows better flow of vital energy and contributes to the effectiveness of acupressure treatments.

Acupuncture

The medical art of acupuncture (from the Latin *acus,* "needle" and *punctura,* a form of the verb "to prick") has been practiced for more than five thousand years by the Chinese. Like acupressure, it is based on the idea of keeping your vital energy in balance. In the place of manual pressure, acupuncture practitioners insert sharp, skinny needles into the skin at acupuncture points along the meridians, like those discussed in "Acupressure" above, in order to unblock obstructed energy.

According to Chinese medicine, diabetes arises from a disharmony or dysfunction of the stomach, spleen, kidney, and lung, and treatment involves restoring normal function to these organ systems. The Chinese also believe diet plays a major role in the management of diabetes and find that patients whose diabetes is well controlled by diet often respond well to acupuncture.

Among people with Type II diabetes, acupuncture may reduce their need for insulin and diabetes pills, but only after prolonged treatment. Acupuncture can relieve pain caused by diabetic neuropathy and may help stimulate functioning of the pancreas, liver, kidneys, and adrenal glands.

How Does Acupuncture Work?

Despite the successful use of acupuncture for thousands of years, Western science has not yet adequately explained or measured how it works. This uncertainty has led some researchers to claim that acupuncture works only because people *believe* it will work. This is referred to as the "placebo effect," but it does not explain why acupuncture relieves pain in animals and infants. Theories regarding its use in pain relief are similar to those previously discussed in "Acupressure." For acupuncture in particular, the endorphin theory is supported by proof of an increased level of endorphins present in the cerebrospinal fluid of people who receive acupuncture treatment. This occurrence may or may not be in synch with the explanation offered by Eastern practitioners: acupuncture and acupressure release blocked vital force along the meridians, which allows for the free flow of energy and the return of the body to a state of balance and harmony.

What to Expect from an Acupuncturist

Acupuncture is not a "do-it-yourself" therapy. Appendix A gives information on how to locate an acupuncturist in your area.

Acupuncture practitioners in the United States usually fall into one of two categories. Western practitioners typically will ask you about your medical history, current treatment program, any complications or symptoms you are experiencing, and then begin treatment. If you go to a medical acupuncturist (an M.D. trained in acupuncture), a physical examination will be conducted as well. There are only about three thousand medical acupuncturists in the United States. For more information, contact the American Academy of Medical Acupuncture (see Appendix A).

The second category of acupuncturists are those who are trained in the traditional Chinese practice. These individuals typically gather information beyond that of the Western practitioners. They observe a person's overall appearance and in particular the eyes, skin, face, and tongue. The Chinese believe the texture, color, and shape of the tongue, for example, can reveal the presence of problems elsewhere in the body. They also gather information about eating habits and elimination problems, and they listen to the voice, breathing, and coughing and note any mouth odor.

Many traditional acupuncturists use a technique called *pulse diagnosis,* which allows them to identify areas in the body that have an energy blockage or disturbance. To accomplish this they feel the radial-artery pulse in the wrist and, from that, check nine different pulses which correspond to different areas of the body. Acupuncturists who are not trained in this method may use an instrument called a *ryodoraku,* which provides similar information. The practitioner will ask you to hold a metal cylinder in the palm of your hand. The acupuncturist then uses a pencillike tool attached to a monitoring device to measure the resistance of specific points along your meridians by touching the *ryodoraku* point to your skin and checking the monitor reading.

Placing the Needles

Acupuncture needles are made of stainless steel or silver alloy and typically are two and a half to three and a half inches long. The practitioner inserts the needles a few millimeters into the skin, where they will remain for about twenty minutes. The exact location and number of needles the practitioner inserts will depend on the condition being treated, although eight to ten needles is a typical amount.

Depending on the practitioner and the nature of your neuropathy, several things may occur once the needles are in place. Some practitioners simply leave the needles untouched until they are removed. If the acupuncturist believes additional stimulation is needed or desired, however, she or he may rotate the needles quickly or slowly in one direction or another. Another technique is electroacupuncture, in which an electric stimulator is attached to the needles to deliver a low-voltage electrical current. According to some practitioners, this technique greatly improves the effectiveness of the treatment.

Does acupuncture hurt? Yes and no. Some people feel little or no pain when the needles are inserted; others say it is a "good hurt," like releasing a tight muscle, or that there is some discomfort at some points but not others. Many people report feeling a pulse of energy flow. After treatment, individuals generally feel more balanced and calm, a state that can last hours to weeks.

Acupuncture for Diabetes

Some points acupuncturists may treat for people with diabetes include the following. Points to treat pain associated with diabetic neuropathy depend on the location of the pain.

- BL 20, located midback on either side of the spine, is a master point for regulating the digestive system.
- BL 21, just below BL 20, regulates the stomach.
- BL 23, on either side of the spine about waist level, is the primary point for regulating kidney function.
- CV 4, located midline on the abdomen below the navel, is key to controlling bladder function, especially with frequent urination.
- KD 5, near the inner ankles, primarily strengthens function of the kidneys.

If you are seeking relief from chronic pain associated with neuropathy, acupuncture often takes effect several days after a treatment. The number of treatments needed will depend on the location and severity of the pain.

Biofeedback

Biofeedback is one of the best examples of a technique that opens up the doors of communication between the mind and body. It is often coupled with visualization or other relaxation methods as a means to achieve overall relief from stress and muscle tension, improve blood circulation, lower blood pressure and blood glucose levels, and relieve pain.

How Does Biofeedback Work?

We receive biofeedback from our bodies every day: we feel hungry when we haven't eaten for a while; when we are under stress, our muscles tense up. These are types of biofeedback we easily recognize. Use of a biofeedback device allows you to become aware of the feedback that occurs on a more subtle level and then use that knowledge to control the functions you want to control and take more responsibility for your health.

To connect with the subtle signals your body sends, you can use a biofeedback electronic monitoring device that measures what's going on physiologically with your body (bio-) and lets you know what that response is (feedback) via some kind of signal, such as beeps or blinking lights or a moving needle on a screen. Typically, these devices have electrodes extending from them, which are placed on the skin over your muscles. The electrodes detect your body's responses and transmit those responses back to the biofeedback machine, which then provides you with information on such body functions as muscle tension, heart rate, skin temperature, blood pressure, and brain waves.

Biofeedback for Diabetes

You can use biofeedback to treat several concerns associated with diabetes. Biofeedback is being used successfully by people with diabetes to improve circulation in their feet and legs. At the University of Wisconsin at La Crosse, for example, forty people used a technique of their choice to relax and then learned biofeedback to increase the blood flow to their toes. Their success is being repeated by people with diabetes all around the United States. When people with diabetes use biofeedback to reduce stress, they experience improved ability to cope with stressful situations, reduced blood glucose levels, and elimination of stress-related symptoms (such as headache, muscle tension, and stomach upset). Biofeedback also can be used to effectively control mild to moderate high blood pressure.

Although you can learn biofeedback at home using home-model biofeedback devices and their accompanying books, it is recommended that you first attend several biofeedback training sessions or treatments so you can learn the procedures firsthand. After initial help from a professional biofeedback therapist (see Appendix A and accompanying box), you may choose to purchase a biofeedback machine for personal use. Many people who learn biofeedback eventually achieve their desired goals without the machine.

For biofeedback to be successful, you need to practice it regularly, even daily, depending on what you hope to achieve. If you are persistent, you will likely succeed. Complement the biofeedback with other forms of relaxation therapy such as breathing therapy, visualization, or meditation, and your chances for success will be very high.

HOW TO CHOOSE A BIOFEEDBACK THERAPIST

• Talk to individuals who are licensed to practice independently or who work under the supervision of a licensed professional. Most biofeedback therapists are also psychologists, nurses, physicians, or other health-care practitioners.

• The Biofeedback Certification Institute of America issues certificates to individuals who pass their high standards for training, experience, and education. Therapists who do not have this certificate may be as well qualified as those who do have one.

• Ask the therapists if they have experience working with people with diabetes. It is recommended that you find someone who is familiar with the disease and its complications.

• Make sure you are comfortable with the therapist. If the individual does not answer your questions fully or you are made to feel ignorant, find another therapist. Poor rapport with the therapist will only increase your stress level.

Bio-Magnetic Touch Healing™

Bio-Magnetic Touch Healing is a new therapeutic technique that uses very light touch to bring about stress reduction and pain relief. There are many touch therapy techniques available that require varying amounts of training, use different levels of touch, and depend on various states of consciousness by the practitioner and the receiver in order to help the body heal itself. Some of these approaches include reiki, SHEN, aura balancing, mahikari, and therapeutic touch. We have chosen to explain Bio-Magnetic Touch Healing for several reasons:

• Perhaps most important, it works, at least according to the many people who have experienced it. After beginning biomagnetic touch, people with diabetes report a reduction in blood glucose levels, better management of their disease, and significantly reduced levels of stress.

• It can be learned easily and effectively by anyone, regardless of age or professional background.

• It takes only a few hours to learn the techniques you need to treat yourself and your family and friends.

• It can be used in conjunction with conventional and other natural healing techniques.

• It is being used by nurses and other health professionals in the U.S., Canada, and other countries, and has been approved by the nurses' associations in several states for continuing education credits.

How Bio-Magnetic Touch Healing Works

Like other touch-therapy techniques, there is no documented scientific evidence to show how or why biomagnetic touch healing works. Certified Bio-Magnetic Touch therapists explain that using light touch on a certain combination of points on the body subtly motivates and activates the body's own healing powers. With repeated treatments, healing continues, and many ailments begin to correct themselves. The result is a body that is in better balance and in more perfect harmony within itself.

Bio-Magnetic Touch Healing for Diabetes

This healing technique is best learned from certified practitioners, who can show you everything from the "Greeting"—a set of points that are touched before any treatment begins, regardless of the reason you are seeking treatment—to points for specific ailments and conditions, including diabetes, neuropathy, hypertension, and heart disease. In just a few hours, you can learn how to treat yourself. (See Appendix A for contact information.) Bio-Magnetic Touch can be done in a few minutes at home, at the office, in your car, or while you're waiting in the dentist's office! A full treatment, however, which balances the entire body, can take thirty minutes or longer.

According to people with diabetes who either receive or give themselves Bio-Magnetic Touch, it has greatly reduced their stress levels, decreased their need for oral diabetes pills, eliminated incidences of hypoglycemia, and improved eyesight. People report better circulation, improved wound healing, and a sense of well-being. Says one gentleman who has had Type II diabetes for seventeen years, "Taking bi-omagnetics makes me feel like I am friends with the whole world."

Breathing Therapy

Breathing is a form of nourishment and can be one of the most effective ways to reduce stress. Most of us don't think about how we breathe unless we have a cold or a condition that makes breathing difficult. So the rest of the time we must be doing it right—right? Wrong. We came into the world knowing how to breathe. As infants we breathed from the diaphragm, which made our belly rise and fall. This is the most natural and healthy way to breathe. As adults we take shallow chest breaths and think we're doing it right.

Before we discuss breathing therapy for diabetes and related complications, we introduce a basic breathing exercise that, with practice, can quickly put you into a state of deep relaxation. Andrew Weil, M.D., one of the world's leading authorities on health and complementary therapies, says that "the single most effective relaxation technique I know is conscious regulation of breath." He recommends the following breathing exercise for everyone. It is an excellent way to start each and every day.

BREATHING EXERCISE

1. Place the tip of your tongue against ridge behind and above the upper front teeth. Keep it there through the entire exercise.
2. Exhale completely through your mouth, making a *whoosh* sound.
3. Inhale deeply and quietly through your nose to the count of four (with mouth closed).
4. Hold your breath for a count of seven.
5. Exhale through your mouth to a count of eight, making a sound.
6. Repeat steps 3, 4, and 5 for a total of four breaths.

You can do this exercise in any position that allows you to inhale and exhale fully. If you are seated, keep your back straight. Practice this breathing technique at least twice a day and whenever you feel stress or the need to focus your thoughts and think more clearly. Do not do more than four breaths at one time during your first month of practice, but you can practice it as often as you wish. After a month, increase to eight breaths each time if you are comfortable with it.

How Does Breathing Therapy Work?

When you practice breathing exercises like those presented in this section, you send nourishment to all the cells of your body. You improve circulation and relieve muscle tension. The result is deep relaxation and often a decrease in blood glucose levels and blood pressure. Deep breathing also strengthens the immune system.

According to many Eastern disciplines, full, deep breathing is essential to health. Deep breathing is recommended as part of your daily routine; practice it while you sit in traffic, during breaks at work, or whenever you feel tense. It can give you an overall surge of energy and vitality every time you do it.

Breathing Therapy for Diabetes

The breathing exercise on page 107 is one you can use for quick pick-me-ups during the day. When you have a little more quiet time, we suggest you try a longer, more concentrated deep-breathing method. Such techniques as the one we explain below can bring your entire body into balance, reduce stress and thus reduce blood glucose levels and hypertension, and allow your energy to flow freely.

To prepare you for the longer breathing exercise, let's begin by learning two breathing techniques: deep breathing and Hara breathing. For both techniques, start from the following position: Lie down on your back with your knees bent or sit in a comfortable chair and loosen any tight clothing. Place your open hands palms down over your abdomen and rib cage so you can feel how they move as you breathe.

The most basic method is **deep breathing.** Take a deep breath; imagine you are a baby and send that breath deep into your abdomen. Feel your belly rise. As your breath moves up into your diaphragm and upper lungs, they, too, will expand. Hold that breath for about three seconds, then slowly exhale. Repeat this cycle several times slowly. Each time concentrate on your breath and the rise and fall of your abdomen, diaphragm, and lungs.

A similar breathing technique is called **Hara breathing.** Take one hand and place it on a spot three finger-widths below your navel. This spot corresponds to an acupressure point known as the "sea of energy" or the Hara. Concentrate on this spot as you breathe deeply into your belly. As you focus on this spot, you will feel your lower abdomen rise and fall as you slowly breathe in and out. This concentrated breathing method helps increase awareness of the body and relieves tension.

You may choose to use breathing therapy to help control stress and blood glucose levels or to relieve pain from diabetic neuropathy. There are several ways to do this, and one way is to combine breathing therapy with visualization. Get into a comfortable position and close your eyes (if you choose). Visualize your breath as a healing force, whatever that is to you—a vibrant light, colors, a flowing river. Concentrate on the area that is painful or tense. As you take a deep breath, send the breath to that area. Imagine that your breath is releasing your tight muscles or easing the pain in that spot. Hold that breath for several seconds and then release it slowly. Visualize your tension or pain leaving as you exhale. Repeat this cycle slowly and comfortably for five to ten minutes.

The following exercise focuses on breathing only and can help relieve pain and stress, stabilize blood glucose levels, and reduce blood pressure. You may want to make a cassette tape of this example so you can use it again and again. (Commercial tapes are also available; see Appendix A.) If you or a friend record it, remember to speak slowly and clearly. The script below is a guide only; you may add to or subtract from it to best suit your needs. Allow five to ten minutes for the exercise, and choose a time and place you will not be disturbed.

Breathe in slowly through your nose to a count of seven. Hold the breath for a second or two. Release the breath slowly and easily. As you breathe out, allow your lips to relax and part slightly and your cheeks to relax. Feel your abdomen fall and your chest relax. Feel the calm that comes with release of your breath.

Breathe in and feel your abdomen expand and rise . . . the rush of breath as it moves easily into your chest.

Feel your chest expand like a balloon and then gently release its air . . . your breath leave through your parted lips. As you exhale, let the breath take any tension in your body with it. Release every molecule of stress and tension into the air with your exhale. As you inhale see yourself becoming more relaxed . . . breathe in relaxation . . . breathe out tension.

Every inhalation sends gentle, soothing breath to every part of your body . . . your feet, your legs, your pelvis, your torso, your hands, your arms, your chest, your face, your head . . . Every inbreath cleanses and releases. Every deep breath brings in more and more peace and quiet.

As you breathe in and out, focus on the Hara, the spot that is three finger-widths below your navel. Breathe into this spot and feel it grow warm. As you breathe in, imagine the Hara opens up and allows any remaining tension or pain in your body to enter. As you exhale, see your tension and pain ride that breath up through your belly, your diaphragm, your lungs. See it leave through your parted lips. As you breathe out, see the tension leave your body.

As you breathe in, feel the warmth radiate from your Hara. Feel it spread to your pelvis and to your hips. As you exhale, feel any tension leave with that breath. Feel the warmth ride with your breath as it leaves your belly, your diaphragm, and your upper chest. With every inbreath, feel the warmth spread into your buttocks and down into your legs and feet. Feel as the breath carries the tension away.

As you inhale, feel your chest wall stretch. Feel your torso gently expand . . . your lower spine open and relax. As you exhale, send out any discomfort. As you inhale, bring in softness and warmth.

Feel each breath as it enters your nose, your throat,

your chest. Every inbreath causes your chin to tilt up slightly as your upper chest moves. As you exhale, your chin settles down slightly. Feel your neck open up to the inbreath; feel your neck settle back when the breath is released. Take a deep breath and feel your shoulders lift up and out slightly. Feel your neck muscles relax. Release the air slowly from your belly, diaphragm, and upper chest.

End your breathing session by taking a complete, slow, deep unifying breath. Feel the breath reach every part of your body and your mind. Allow the breath to penetrate every corner of your being. Hold it for several seconds and then release it slowly. Release all tension. Allow in peace and calm.

Whenever possible, take a few minutes to breathe in a healthy, relaxing way. If you don't always have time for the longer exercise above, do the brief exercise at the beginning of this section. Every deep breath you take can bring you closer to a relaxed state and better control of your diabetes.

Herbal Medicine

Herbs were our ancient ancestors' first line of defense against illness and disease, and in many places in the world, they are still very much a part of healing. From the ancient Greeks to the Chinese to Native Americans, practitioners of herbal medicine have been scorned, murdered, and admired over the millennia as our understanding of the power of plants has grown. Today there is a resurgent interest in the use of herbs to heal people with various ailments and conditions. Diabetes and many of its complications are among them.

According to the World Health Organization, up to 80 percent of the people in the world use herbal remedies.

Although the percentage of people in the United States in that category is significantly lower, for a growing number of them herbs, along with diet, are becoming the treatment of choice for many ailments. For a serious, chronic disease such as diabetes, herbs can play a complementary role, augmenting the healing powers of diet, exercise, and stress management. Some of the herbs useful for treating diabetes and its complications may be in your kitchen at this very moment. Garlic and onion, for example, have both been proven to be important in treating heart disease. The spice fenugreek is used around the world in treating diabetes.

Before we continue, one note of caution: *Do not use any herbs or herbal formulas without first checking with your physician.* Herbs can interact with other medications you may be taking, and some have a significant effect on blood glucose levels, blood pressure, and body functions. Monitor your blood glucose levels when taking herbs to gauge their effect. Consult a knowledgeable herbalist and share his or her recommendations with your diabetes management team.

How Herbal Medicine Works

Herbs contain a myriad of active compounds, such as enzymes, vitamins, proteins, and sugars, that work together in unique ways to produce healing qualities that are special for each plant. When you take an herb that has properties specific for your ailment or condition, these compounds interact with compounds in your body to treat your symptoms and restore your vital energy. Nature ''knows'' what works.

Herbalists will prescribe either a single herb or a combination to create a complete herbal remedy that is specific for your needs. Some of these single and combination herbals are available through commercial herbal manufacturers; others are prepared by herbalists. Both base their formulas on those that have been handed down through many cultures and many centuries.

Since ancient times, the perception among those who use herbs has been that disease results when there is an imbalance or lack of harmony within the body; and that natural healing will occur when an individual's physical, spiritual, and emotional states regain their balance. Herbs carry the messages of harmony and balance to the body as they heal.

Choosing Herbal Remedies for Diabetes and Its Complications

We have learned a great deal from many cultures about the use of herbs for diabetes, especially from the Native Americans. Diabetes was rare among them until they were introduced to the Western diet. Now Native Americans have the highest incidence of the disease in the world. Their indigenous diet contained many plant foods that were insulin analogs (having functions similar to those of insulin). Some of those plants are included in the following list.

This alphabetical list of herbs is for treatment of diabetes and some of its complications, such as hypertension, poor circulation, pain (neuropathy), retinopathy, glaucoma, and cataracts. Most herbs have several uses, yet here we describe only the ones that relate to diabetes and associated conditions. See the box "Types of Herbal Formulas," pp. 121–22, for help on choosing the right herbal formulation.

Alfalfa *(Medicago sativa)*
Part Used: Leaves
Uses: Often a food of the Native Americans, alfalfa helps lower blood cholesterol levels.
Dose: Pour one pint of boiling water over one ounce of the leaves. Let steep for five to twenty minutes. Drink hot or warm, one to two cups per day, upon wakening and retiring.

NOTE: In animal studies, alfalfa has retarded the development of streptozotocin diabetes (see Chapter 1).

Bilberry *(Vaccinium myrtillus)*
Part Used: Fruit
Uses: Bilberry fruit can reduce blood glucose levels. This herb is also known for its effectiveness in improving vision. It is available as a tincture, in concentrated drops, and in capsules and tablets.
Dose: Prepare as an infusion using one teaspoon of dried berries in one cup of water. Drink one cup per day. For commercial formulations, take according to label directions.
NOTE: Bilberry is completely nontoxic even when taken at high doses for an extended time.

Bitter melon *(Momordica charantia)*
Part Used: Fruit
Uses: This tropical fruit has been used as a folk medicine for diabetes in many cultures. The fresh juice or extract of the ripe bitter melon lowers blood glucose levels. Bitter melon contains charantin, a hypoglycemic agent that is more potent than the oral hypoglycemic drug tolbutamide, as well as an insulinlike protein that reduces blood glucose levels when injected into people with Type I diabetes.
Dose: Two ounces of the juice per day.
NOTE: The juice is extremely bitter.

Burdock *(Arctium lappa)*
Part Used: Root
Uses: This common weed, eaten as a vegetable by the Native Americans, may help lower blood glucose levels. It is high in inulin, an insulin analog. It also increases kidney function and urine output and is a general tissue cleanser.
Dose: To make a decoction, add one teaspoon of root (one-

year-old roots or younger only) to twenty-four ounces of boiling water. Steep for thirty minutes. Drink at room temperature, one to two cups daily.

NOTE: The taste is sweet with a slight bitter edge.

Cayenne *(Capsicum frutescens)*
Part Used: Fruit

Uses: Also known as the common chili pepper, this herb contains a compound called capsaicin, which is used to alleviate nerve pain (neuropathy) associated with diabetes.

Dose: Topical applications of capsaicin cream, as needed, for pain.

NOTE: Side effects are limited and mild and may include some skin irritation.

Fenugreek *(Trigonella foenumgraecum)*
Part Used: Seeds

Uses: The seeds of this legume and spice contain alkaloids trigonelline and cumarin, which help reduce glucose levels in urine, improve glucose tolerance, and significantly reduce cholesterol levels in Type II diabetes. Fenugreek is available as a powder, tablet, capsule, and an extract.

Dose: To prepare an infusion, place two teaspoons of seeds in 1 cup of water and let stand for five hours. Boil for one minute. Drink two to three cups per day.

NOTE: Do not use during pregnancy, as it can stimulate uterine contractions. Fenugreek is available as a powder, tablet, capsule, an extract, and as concentrated drops.

Garlic *(Allium sativum)*
Part Used: Cloves ·

Uses: Garlic and its relative the onion *(Allium cepa)* help reduce blood glucose levels. These plants contain sulfur compounds that have chemical structures similar to those of insulin, and these compounds—allicin and allyl propyl disulphide—are believed to lower glucose levels. Garlic also lowers cholesterol, triglyceride, and low-density lipoprotein cholesterol levels while increasing high-density lipoprotein cholesterol levels. Garlic is available in powder, tablet, capsules, and liquid. Fresh uncooked garlic is the best way to reap its benefits.

Dose: One clove (three grams of fresh or one gram of dried) per day; or one-half teaspoon of the juice three times daily. Take commercial products according to package directions.

Ginkgo *(Ginkgo biloba)*
Part Used: Leaves
Uses: Ginkgo—the oldest living tree species—aids in protecting the health of the capillaries and improves blood flow, especially in medium and small arteries. It is available in tablets, concentrated drops, tinctures, extracts, and capsules.

Dose: As an infusion, use one-half ounce of leaves to one pint of water. Pour boiling water over the leaves and steep for five to twenty minutes. Drink hot or warm, one to two cups a day, upon wakening and at bedtime. Take commercial formulations according to package directions.
NOTE: Buy a ginkgo extract standardized to contain 24 percent ginkgo flavoglycosides. Take forty milligrams three times per day.

Ginseng, Siberian *(Eleutherococcus senticosus)*
Part Used: Root
Uses: Siberian ginseng can aid in regulation and reduction of blood glucose levels. It helps the body adapt to stress, including the stress caused by blood glucose fluctuations, improves mood, and helps in weight loss.

Dose: For a decoction, add one-half teaspoon of powdered root to one cup of hot water. Drink in the morning, at lunch, and at bedtime.

NOTE: Siberian ginseng rarely causes adverse side effects. There are many products claiming to contain Siberian ginseng that actually do not. Only buy from reputable companies.

Green tea (various species)

Part Used: Leaves

Uses: In addition to its reported anticancer effects, green tea also helps keep serum cholesterol levels low. It is available as a tea and in capsules.

Dose: For an infusion, add one pint of boiling water to 1 ounce of leaves. Steep for five to twenty minutes and drink hot or warm, one to two cups per day, upon wakening and at bedtime.

NOTE: Because green tea contains caffeine, you may want to steep the leaves for only two to three minutes to keep the caffeine levels low—it has twenty to thirty milligrams of caffeine per cup.

Gymnema *(Gymnema sylvestre)*

Part Used: Leaves

Uses: This member of the milkweed family is useful in both Type I and II diabetes. It has been used by Ayurvedic healers for diabetes for two thousand years. Studies in the early 1990s suggest that dried gymnema or gymnema extract may repair or regenerate the beta cells in the pancreas, which in turn increases blood insulin levels. Gymnema also decreases triglyceride and cholesterol levels, and can assist in losing weight by taking the edge off of your sweet tooth and creating feelings of satiety.

Dose: Use four hundred milligrams per day of the extract.

NOTE: Unlike oral hypoglycemic drugs, gymnema lowers

blood glucose levels in diabetics only; it has no effect on healthy individuals. It has no known toxic effects.

Hawthorn *(Crataegus oxycantha)*
Parts Used: Flowers, leaves, and berries
Uses: Hawthorn is used widely as a heart remedy, as it lowers peripheral resistance to blood flow.
Dose: Pour one pint of boiling water over one teaspoon of flowers and steep for five to twenty minutes. Drink one to two cups daily, a mouthful at a time. It is available commercially as an extract: take 100 to 250 milligrams three times daily.
NOTE: No reported cases of toxic reactions. Combined with motherwort, it may prove to be effective in preventing or treating atherosclerosis. It takes about two weeks for hawthorn's blood-pressure-lowering effect to take place.

Nettle *(Urtica dioica)*
Parts Used: Roots, leaves, and seeds
Uses: Nettle can lower the amount of glucose in the blood.
Dose: One teaspoon of granulated leaves or root per cup of boiling water. Drink cold, one tablespoon at a time, one cup per day.
NOTE: The green tops of the plant are an excellent source of nutrients and can be added, boiled, to soups.

Oat Straw *(Avena sativa)*
Part Used: Straw
Uses: Oat straw can significantly lower blood cholesterol, which helps combat heart disease. It also lowers blood glucose levels.
Dose: One to two teaspoons, once a day, mixed in food or a beverage.
NOTE: Can reduce blood cholesterol levels by 20 percent.

Raspberry, Red *(Rubus* spp.*)*
Part Used: Leaves
Uses: Red raspberry leaves help control high blood glucose levels and promote insulin production.
Dose: For an infusion, add one teaspoon of the leaf in one cup of boiling water. Drink cold, one to two cups per day. If pregnant, steep one-half ounce with one pint of boiling water for three to five minutes. Drink warm, one pint per day.
NOTE: Raspberry infusions are also good for the symptoms of morning sickness.

Wood Betony *(Betonica officinalis)*
Part Used: Leaves
Uses: Wood betony contains trigonelline, which reportedly lowers blood glucose levels.
Dose: Pour one pint of water over one ounce of leaves and allow to steep for five to twenty minutes. Drink hot or warm, one to two cups or more per day.
NOTE: Wood betony is also effective in relieving depression, tension, and anxiety.

Chinese Herbs for Diabetes

The Chinese have a long history of treating chronic conditions such as diabetes with herbal remedies. According to tradition, the Chinese prepare their herbal remedies by decoction, but their approach is slightly different from the one explained in the "Types of Herbal Formulas" box in this section. You can purchase Chinese herbs at an Oriental grocery store or health food store.

To prepare a decoction using Chinese herbs, place the prescribed amount of herb in an earthenware pot. Add cold water until the herb is covered and then add eight ounces more. Stir and let the herbs soak for about twenty minutes. Keep the pot covered. Bring the mixture to a boil. Once the water boils, reduce the heat and simmer for ten to twenty minutes, depending on how heavy the herbs are. Roots and stems, for example, need to simmer longer than do leaves. Cool the decoction to a comfortable temperature before drinking. The Chinese usually drink one to two cups twice a day. Children younger than fourteen years should take half that amount.

Chouwutong *(Clerodendron trichotomum thunb)*
Parts Used: Young branches and leaves
Uses: This herb helps reduce blood pressure and also has pain-relieving qualities.
Dose: Two to four teaspoons.
NOTE: This herb has an offensive odor.

Huangjing *(Polygonatum kingianum)*
Part Used: Rhizome
Uses: Huangjing can reduce blood glucose and blood fat levels as well as reduce blood pressure.
Dose: Two to four teaspoons.
NOTE: This is a sticky herb, so it needs to be decocted a bit longer in order to release its active ingredients.

Shanyao *(Dioscorea opposita thunb)*
Part Used: Tuberous root
Uses: Reduces blood glucose levels.
Dose: Use one tablespoon.
NOTE: This sweet herb also tones the kidneys.

Shudihuang *(Rehmannia glutinosa libosch)*
Part Used: Tuberous root
Uses: This sweet herb is used to tone up the blood and reduce blood glucose levels.
Dose: Four teaspoons.

NOTE: Shudihuang also helps tone the kidneys and protect the liver.

Where to Get Herbs

Herbal remedies are made from the root, bulb, stem, bark, flower, fruit, seed, resin, or rhizome of herbs, leafy plants, weeds, ferns, trees, or lichens. You can get herbs either from your herbalist; at commercial outlets such as health or natural food stores, homeopathic pharmacies, or through a naturopath or mail order house; or you can grow and dry your own. Appendix B lists some mail order outlets for herbs. If you want to grow and dry your own herbs, refer to the Bibliography and Suggested Reading or consult with an herbalist in your area.

TYPES OF HERBAL FORMULAS

Herbal preparations come in several forms. Many are available over the counter as tablets or capsules; others can be purchased as a tea or a liquid. You may choose to prepare your own remedies from herbs you dry yourself or dried herbs you purchase from an herb store or herbalist. Below are basic instructions on how to prepare infusions, extracts, and decoctions. Glass or earthenware pots are preferred over metal for preparing these formulas.

Infusions are made from the leaves, flowers, or other soft parts of a plant. They are prepared like teas, only they use more of the herb than other teas and they steep longer for greater potency.

To prepare an infusion, pour two cups of boiling water over two to three tablespoons of the herb and steep for at least ten minutes or even overnight in the refrigerator in a tightly covered pot. Strain the liquid. Drink the infusion hot, warm, or cool, depending on the herb and the effect you want. Herbal infusions decompose rapidly, so make a fresh batch daily and keep it cool. If you are not used to herbal teas, these formulas may taste a bit unusual to you. Add lemon, fruit juice, or artificial sweeteners for taste if desired.

Decoctions are prepared from the roots, stems, and bark of herbs. To prepare a standard decoction, boil one ounce of herb in one pint of water in a covered nonmetallic container for twenty to thirty minutes. Strain the liquid and cool. Doses vary from one teaspoon to one cup taken three to six times a day. Decoctions also deteriorate rapidly and should be made fresh and kept refrigerated for no more than a day or two.

Extracts are stronger than infusions and are preferred by practitioners because they have a higher concentration of active ingredients. You can purchase commercially made extracts through many health and nutrition stores, pharmacies, herbalists, other natural health practitioners, and mail order. If you want to make your own, the simplest preparation is a green extract made by thoroughly crushing the juicy parts of the plant and pressing out the juices. For medicinal purposes, one ounce of extract equals one ounce of the pure dry herb. Extracts deteriorate rapidly, so make fresh batches as needed.

GUIDELINES FOR HERBAL USE

• When used properly, herbal remedies are very safe. As with any substance, however, misuse or abuse may cause unwanted side effects. Seek the advice of a knowledgeable herbalist, naturopath, or homeopath to help you select the herbal remedies that are best for you. Refer to Appendix A and the Suggested Reading List for more information.

• Some herbs interact with prescription and over-the-counter drugs as well as with other herbs. If you are taking insulin, diabetes pills, or any other conventional drugs, check with a physician, herbalist, or pharmacist who is familiar with both the pharmacology of herbs and of your medications before you taken an herbal remedy. The manufacturers of herbal remedies and their staff researchers also should be able to answer your questions over the telephone.

• Some people feel nauseous if they take herbs on an empty stomach. To avoid this, take your remedy after you have eaten a meal or snack.

• If you experience nausea, diarrhea, or any other unexpected symptom after taking an herb, stop taking it and call your herbalist or physician. You may need to switch to a different remedy.

• Some people prefer to use fresh, freeze-dried herbs because they claim they contain more of the plant's active ingredients than those which are processed traditionally. Experts have not substantiated this claim as of yet.

Homeopathy

Homeopathy (*homeo,* like; *pathos,* disease) is a system of medicine in which the remedies stimulate the body's internal healing energies so it can heal itself. It is based on the concept that "like may be cured by like," which means the remedies prescribed by homeopaths—those who practice homeopathy—are capable of producing the primary symptoms you are already experiencing. If this sounds like exactly what you don't want to happen, don't worry. During its two-hundred-year history, homeopathy has been used successfully around the world for a wide variety of medical conditions, including chronic diseases such as diabetes.

There are approximately two thousand homeopathic remedies, but only about one hundred to two hundred are used regularly. Most remedies are derived from plants; the rest are made from minerals or animal substances. Several remedies can be used to treat diabetes or help prevent diabetic symptoms or complications associated with the disease, such as hypertension, glaucoma, cataracts, and blood vessel disease.

How Homeopathic Remedies Work

Unlike allopathic (conventional) medicine, which works on a physical level, homeopathy is an energy medicine. Like acupuncture, it works with the body's vital energy to promote healing. The natural tendency of the vital force is health and balance, and homeopathic remedies allow the force to achieve that goal in a unique way.

Homeopaths prescribe remedies based on a substance's ability to allow the cause of a symptom to resolve itself. They do this by choosing a remedy which, if consumed in a normal or large quantity, will cause the same symptoms they want to eliminate. However, the dose they prescribe will contain only a very minute amount—or perhaps not even a trace—of the remedy. That's because in homeopathy, *remedies are the most potent the more they are diluted.* That is, less is more.

This sounds unusual, but it's true. To make a homeopathic remedy, one drop of the base formula—the chosen plant part—is mixed with ninety-nine drops of water or alcohol. This is shaken well and then one drop of this mixture is added to ninety-nine drops of water or alcohol and shaken again. This process, called *potentization,* is repeated again and again, perhaps hundreds of times. Although it seems the formulation should become weaker and more ineffective each time it is diluted, *the opposite is true. The more times a remedy goes through potentization, the greater is its potency.*

Scientists have not yet found the reason this is so. Some experts favor the quantum physics theory, which explains it this way: All physical substances are composed of energy, and when they move or change position, they leave an energy field behind them, like footsteps in the sand. During repeat potentization, the resulting remedies may not contain any molecules of the original substance, yet the molecules' "footsteps" are there. These footsteps exist at high energy levels, and thus result in a high-potency remedy.

HOW TO TAKE HOMEOPATHIC REMEDIES

Homeopathic remedies are available from your practitioner, at a drug or health food store, or mail order (see Appendix B). If you want to make your own remedies, consult with a homeopath or see Suggested Reading for a list of books that can help you.

Homeopathic remedies are typically available as drops or tablets (sugar pills) that have been infused with the remedy. These remedies are prepared by homeopathic pharmacies according to the guidelines of the *Homeopathic Pharmacopoeia of the United States,* the official manufacturing manual recognized by the Food and Drug Administration.

• At least ten but preferably thirty minutes before taking a remedy, do not put anything into your mouth, including food, beverages, gum, mouthwash, toothpaste, or tobacco smoke.

• Avoid taking conventional medicine, such as aspirin, ibuprofen, or laxatives while using a homeopathic remedy. If you are using insulin or diabetes pills, consult with your physician before you start the homeopathic remedy.

• Homeopathic drops and tablets are dissolved on or under the tongue so absorption can occur through the mucous membranes of the mouth. You don't need to wash them down with water.

• Coffee can cancel the benefits of many remedies. Avoid coffee, regular or decaffeinated, while on a course of homeopathic treatment.

Homeopathy for Diabetes

Diabetes is a chronic disease, and as such is more deeply seated than an acute condition, such as the flu or bronchitis. That does not mean homeopathy has no role in treating diabetes. *We do recommend, however, that you work closely with your homeopath and your management team if you choose homeopathic treatment.*

Dr. Andrew Lockie, author of *The Family Guide to Homeopathy,* recommends a *constitutional* remedy in addition to conventional treatment for diabetes. A constitutional remedy is broad based and serves to stimulate your body's physical and mental healing powers. Constitutional remedies work at a deep level and gradually help strengthen the vital force. This strengthening process can decrease the frequency and severity of any acute symptoms you may experience, such as hypoglycemia, and help reduce or prevent complications associated with diabetes.

Your homeopath will choose a constitutional remedy specifically for you, based on information gathered during your visit. This information includes your current physical and emotional state, an assessment of your personality, your hopes and fears, and your family history. The homeopath may also ask you questions you may think are unusual, such as "Do your hands and feet get cold often?" and "Do you walk or talk in your sleep?" It is essential to have a complete picture of your physical, emotional, and spiritual state—the mind/body—in order to choose the best remedy for you. Much of what homeopaths learn is done by listening to you and observing your behavior and even how you dress. If the homeopath suspects an underlying condition, he or she may ask you to undergo medical tests. Until you and your homeopath have identified a constitutional treatment for you, she or he may prescribe another remedy to relieve symptoms you may be experiencing.

Many homeopathic remedies have been applied to the treatment of diabetes and its complications. Homeopathic remedies generally do not make it possible to reduce the use of insulin or diabetes pills, yet according to Dana Ullman, author of *The Consumer's Guide to Homeopathy* and several other books on the subject, some people with diabetes who take homeopathic remedies do reduce their insulin requirements and have enjoyed an improvement in pancreatic function. In any case, homeopathic remedies can improve overall health and symptoms associated with diabetes. Although homeopathic remedies are safe, *do not attempt to self-treat with homeopathy without consulting your physician and a homeopath who can guide your choice of remedies and dosing.*

Dosing

Perhaps you have seen homeopathic remedies in your pharmacy. If you were to look at the label for, say, belladonna, you might see: "Belladonna 30c 2h." What does this mean? The "30c" is the potency, or strength, of the remedy. The higher the number, the greater the strength of the remedy. Thus 30c is more potent than 6c, which is another common potency. The *c* refers to the centesimal scale, which is how the remedy was diluted. The centesimal scale is the most commonly used system in the United States, and the 6c and 30c dosages are the most widely prescribed. To appreciate how potent a 30c dose is, a 1c remedy is diluted 1:100; a 2c, 1:10,000, and so on. The *2h* on the label means take the remedy every two hours.

How potent a remedy is and how often you should take it are highly individual and depend on your particular needs, your homeopath, and the manufacturer of the remedy. The ultimate goal of any remedy, however, is always the same: to gently stimulate your own healing process to restore balance and health.

A few words about dosing of homeopathic remedies before we introduce some remedies to you:

• Remedies are chosen for the individual. Therefore two people with Type II diabetes probably will not be prescribed the same remedy.

• Most homeopaths prescribe a single remedy at a time. If one does not bring relief, they will ask you to stop taking that one and prescribe another.

• Always follow the dosages prescribed by your homeopath or the ones stated on the label. If you don't notice any improvement or you have questions about the remedy, consult a homeopath or homeopathic pharmacist.

• Occasionally, a remedy may make you feel worse before it makes you feel better. This temporary flare-up in symptoms, called proving, indicates that a particular remedy is working. Depending on the symptom, the flare-up may last only a few minutes. Not everyone experiences these reactions. Proving may occur if the potency you took was too high for you. Consult with a homeopath or try a lower potency.

• Once your symptoms begin to improve, stop the remedy. If, however, the improvement does not continue or you begin to feel worse again, restart the remedy at a higher potency. If your worsening symptoms are accompanied by confusion, fever, or other new symptoms, contact your homeopath or physician immediately.

Remedies

The following list of remedies gives you a starting point from which to begin your exploration of homeopathy and what it can offer you.

Aconite *(Aconitum napellus)* is made from an herb and is used to treat acute glaucoma. It is also effective in treating pain associated with neuropathy, as it depresses the sensory nerve endings. Aconite is fast acting and works best if taken at the first sign of symptoms. Individuals who respond best to aconite are usually energetic and may look nervous or anxious. They often crave cold liquids and may have hot, red faces.

Arnica *(Arnica montana)* is derived from an herb and is used to treat diabetic retinitis (inflammation of the retina). This remedy causes improvement in the central blood flow to the eyes. Arnica is indicated in individuals who feel thirsty, restless, or to whom everything they lie on feels too hard.

Carbo vegetabilis is derived from the charcoal of beech, birch, or poplar wood. It is used in individuals who have poor circulation to the hands and feet caused by diabetes or arteriosclerosis. This remedy is most effective in people who feel mentally sluggish and who have patchy memory, a craving for sweets and salty foods, and have dry mouth in the morning.

Gelsemium *(Gelsemium sempervirens)* is prepared from the roots of this plant and is a very useful remedy for glaucoma, especially in those experiencing double vision and when the eyes feel bruised and under pressure. It is also indicated for people with hypertension who feel dizzy and weak. Individuals who respond best to gelsemium are generally mentally and physically sluggish and feel drowsy.

Graphites is a mixture of carbon, iron, and silica. It is helpful in poor wound healing, cramps in the hands and feet, and constipation. You are most likely to be helped by graphites if you are overweight, elderly, and a woman; or if you have coarse features, dark hair, and an earthy complexion. People who do hard manual labor outside or who drive heavy vehicles also benefit from graphites.

Natrum muriaticum is derived from common salt, sodium chloride. It has several uses for complications associated with diabetes. It is useful for cataracts, especially in individuals who have a history of excessive salt intake. Symptoms of cataracts include hazy, misty vision that improves in dimly lit areas. It is also one of the basic remedies for hypertension, as it promotes relaxation and helps eliminate excessive fluid retention. Natrum muriaticum also can help relieve the need to urinate frequently.

Characteristics of individuals who are helped by natrum muriaticum include people who have a squarish build and who walk on their heels, have sandy or dark hair, and greasy skin. They often are very thirsty, tend to be constipated, and have acne.

Nux vomica *(Strychnos nux-vomica)* is made from the dried, ripe seeds of the poison-nut tree. This remedy helps people with diabetes who are experiencing stupor and vertigo, buzzing in the ears, insomnia, or having feelings of anger, frustration, anxiety, and hopelessness. Individuals who respond best to nux vomica are usually self-reliant, workaholic, nervous, and irritable. Many are thin, prematurely bald, and often have indigestion.

Phosphoric acid works primarily on the nervous system and is often used in early-stage diabetes. It works best in nervous individuals who have a mild, yielding temperament and, among children, those who are gangly and thin. Phosphoric acid can alleviate apathy; difficulty in understanding what is going on; headaches that are made worse by noise; debility and bruised feeling in muscles; symptoms worsened by grief, worry, anxiety.

Phosphorus is made from white phosphorus and is most

helpful in people who are eliminating large amounts of urine and who are restless and have dry mouth and dry skin. Adults who respond well to phosphorus are usually tall, well proportioned, have fine skin, or have dark or fair skin with copper highlights in their hair. They exhibit lots of vitality that alternates with sudden tiredness, and they are often hungry because of their rapid metabolism. In children it works best in those who are tall and thin.

One advantage of homeopathic remedies is that, unlike drugs, they do not cause side effects. They do require some patience, however. If you take a remedy for an acute symptom and you do not get some improvement after a few doses, you should try another remedy. If you take a constitutional remedy, you will be building overall strength of your vital force, and changes may be subtle.

Homeopathic remedies also are less expensive than most traditional drugs. They are easy to administer and have either a sweet or a slight taste. When you follow the directions of your physician or those on the label, they are a safe, effective complement to conventional medical treatments.

Hypnosis

There's a common misconception that people who are hypnotized can be "made" to perform ridiculous tricks or behaviors against their will. Hypnosis is about having control, not about losing it. It is a state of intense concentration, an altered state of awareness—not a loss of free will or consciousness—in which individuals have an increased ability to respond to suggestions presented by another person or by themselves. As a form of therapy, hypnosis is used to treat a variety of conditions, but much of its success is in relieving stress. Ninety-four percent of people who undergo hypnosis induced by themselves or another person benefit from the experience, even if relaxation is the only advantage they receive.

Karen Olness, M.D., professor of pediatrics at the Case Western Reserve Medical Center in Cleveland and an expert in hypnotherapy, reports that people use hypnosis to stabilize their blood glucose levels, while Martin Rossman, M.D., clinical associate professor of medicine at the University of California's San Francisco Medical Center, has patients who control blood pressure through hypnosis. In this section we focus on how you can use hypnosis, specifically self-hypnosis, to reduce stress and tension and, in turn, stabilize your blood glucose and blood-pressure levels. Although not addressed specifically here, hypnosis also can be used to relieve pain associated with diabetic neuropathy. (See Bibliography and Suggested Reading.)

If you prefer to have someone hypnotize you, refer to Appendix A for information on how to contact professional hypnotherapists. If you would like to learn self-hypnosis, you have several choices. You can learn through a book, audiotape, or videotape; information is included in Appendix A. However, we recommend you learn through individual lessons with a professional hypnotherapist until you know enough to do it on your own. Self-hypnosis is much more useful—and inexpensive—than returning again and again to a hypnotherapist. Once you learn self-hypnosis, you can practice it anytime.

How Does Hypnosis Work?

In hypnosis, you deliberately divert your attention away from some aspect of yourself, such as emotional upset, physical pain, or muscle tension, and concentrate on some type of imagery. The act of focusing your attention places you in an altered state of awareness. Brain-wave studies show that people who are in a hypnotic state have reduced brain-wave patterns, indicating a sleeplike state. The secret of hypnosis, however, is not just being in an altered state of awareness but in how you use that hypnotic state to improve some aspect of your health or behavior. This leaves the list of possible uses for hypnosis wide open: you can reduce stress, lose weight, lower your blood pressure, stabilize your glucose levels, and even motivate yourself to exercise!

Self-Hypnosis for Diabetes: Autogenic Training

Many people go to a hypnotherapist to be trained in self-hypnosis so they have the freedom to control their stress levels and stabilize their diabetes themselves. One form of self-hypnosis is called autogenic training, which was developed by Dr. Johannes Schultz in 1929. The goal of autogenic training is the sense "I am at peace." This state of altered awareness can be reached by silently repeating different phrases while you concentrate on the body part that corresponds to the phrase.

You may want to experience a group autogenic-training session taught by a certified instructor, or you can receive individual instruction. Many people learn autogenics from self-help books (see Bibliography and Suggested Reading). The autogenic procedure described below is a standard one. Read over the following guidelines before you start.

• Choose a comfortable, quiet location where you will not be disturbed for at least twenty-five to thirty minutes. The first few times you try this technique, it may take you up to fifteen minutes to fully enter a hypnotic state and focus on your goals. Once you are adept at relaxing and entering a trance, your entire session can last as little as eight to ten minutes.

• "Should I sit or lie down?" It's your choice; do what is most comfortable for you.

• "Should I close my eyes?" Many people close them once they are in a hypnotic state because it helps them visualize and focus more clearly. If keeping your eyes open works for you, do it.

• Proper breathing is essential. Refer to "Breathing Therapy" for guidelines on deep breathing. Do the short breathing exercise at the beginning of the section and then proceed with the exercise below.

As you complete the breathing exercise, continue to breathe easily and peacefully. As you breathe, repeat silently the phrase "I am at peace" until you reach a state of relaxation.

Once you feel relaxed, repeat silently, "My right arm is heavy." Repeat it several times while concentrating on your right arm. Observe how your right arm feels and notice any emotions or feelings that arise as you focus on your arm. There is no right or wrong way to feel; simply feel. If any other thoughts come to mind, allow them to leave and refocus on your arm.

Repeat silently, "My left arm is heavy." Again, repeat it several times while concentrating on your left arm and observe any emotions or feelings.

Do the same procedure for each of the following phrases:

"My right leg is heavy."
"My left leg is heavy."
"My arms and legs are heavy and warm."
"Heartbeat calm and regular."
"Breathing calm and regular."
"My center is warm."
"My forehead is cool."
"My neck and shoulders are heavy."
"I am _____ (give a personal affirmation, such as "I feel peace and lightness in my heart," or "I am at peace with my diabetes").

It is best to do this autogenic exercise twice a day for about twenty minutes each time. Once you master entering a hypnotic state quickly, you can probably do a session in fifteen minutes or less, enough time to do it on your break at work. This simple technique can regulate blood and energy flow, relieve stress and tension, and help you relax completely.

ARE YOU A CANDIDATE FOR HYPNOSIS?

Will self-hypnosis work for you? Read the following statements. If you can answer yes to each of them, chances are good that hypnosis will work for you.

- *I have a good imagination.* This includes all your senses. Most people have a vivid imagination, yet some don't believe they do. For hypnosis to work it's important that you believe in your power of imagination.
- *I want to take personal responsibility for my health.* Whether you are taking insulin, diabetes pills, or other medications to control complications of diabetes, you have handed over control of your health to drugs. Some of these medications may be necessary, but self-hypnosis may help you take back at least some control. This requires a firm commitment to learn the technique.
- *I know exactly what I want out of self-hypnosis.* Set realistic goals and believe in them. You may want to reduce your dependence on insulin or eliminate use of diabetes pills. How will you do that? Perhaps you want to lose weight or stabilize your blood glucose levels. Maybe you're more interested in improving circulation to your feet or relieving pain caused by neuropathy. Define your goals clearly so your attention will be focused on them.
- *I am willing to dedicate the time it takes to learn self-hypnosis.* Self-hypnosis is not a quick-fix therapy, and

> there are no self-hypnosis pills. It usually requires weeks, and sometimes months, of daily practice. Those who stick with it are usually glad they did.

Hypnosis is a fascinating therapy and is of special interest to people with diabetes because it places the reins of control entirely in the hands of the individual. Although the path to that control will take time and commitment on your part, the rewards can be very fulfilling.

Massage

When you hear the word *massage,* how many different varieties come to mind? If you said five or ten, or even fifty, you'd be off by a long shot. According to a survey published in *The New England Journal of Medicine,* there are about one hundred different types of massage. Deep tissue, Esalen, Hawaiian, Oriental, sport, Swedish, Thai, Touch for Health—these are just a few of the massage techniques from which you can choose.

In simple terms, massage is the manipulation of the body's soft tissues, using strokes that knead, tap, vibrate, and glide, among other motions, for therapeutic purposes. Below, we explain two of the most popular massage techniques with which people in the United States are most familiar and which can be helpful for people with diabetes. One is Swedish massage (also called Western or traditional massage), during which oil is applied to the entire body and various stroke techniques are used to work the soft tissues. Another popular type of massage is Oriental massage, which, unlike the Swedish variety, does not involve the use of oil and does not require you to remove your clothing. There are some other basic differences between these two approaches, which we discuss below. Also see the Bibliography and Suggested Reading for more information on these and other massage techniques.

CAUTION: Your physician may recommend that massage of your legs be avoided, as it could further stress your blood vessels. Leg massage should also be avoided if you have varicose veins or phlebitis. People with high fever, vomiting, nausea, diarrhea, jaundice, cancer, or bleeding should avoid full-body massage.

Oriental Massage

Oriental massage is based solely on the premise that massage moves and balances the vital force, or chi in the Chinese tradition. Oriental massage promotes the free flow of the vital force through the body by unblocking areas where it has become congested. Oriental massage is effective in relieving overall tension, improving circulation, and lowering high blood pressure.

How Does Oriental Massage Work?

As the Oriental massage practitioner stimulates the free flow of vital force through your body, this process returns your body to balance and promotes healing. There are two basic approaches to Oriental massage. One is called *amma,* in which gentle strokes, rubbing, kneading, and mild pressure are used to relieve simple stress and tension and gently stimulate blood circulation. An amma session lasts about an hour. The other method is called *tui na,* in which practitioners gently but vigorously rub, tap, press, push, squeeze, twist, and roll the muscles to move the vital force. This slightly more aggressive approach is considered to be more "problem oriented" than *amma* because it works at a deeper level in the body. *Tui na* helps promote blood circulation, lower blood pressure, stimulate organ functioning, and treat stiff joints. It is usually performed very rapidly, with a session lasting about twenty to thirty minutes.

Of key importance in Oriental massage, unlike Swedish massage, is the special connection between you and the practitioner. As Oriental massage therapists massage the points along your meridian lines, they focus on each point and concentrate on connecting their consciousness and energy with yours. According to Oriental massage tradition, this mind/body connection is critical for healing to occur.

Both the *amma* and *tui na* approaches to Oriental massage ''wake up'' the energy at your pressure points, which in turn promotes blood circulation, enhances nerve health, and leaves you feeling revitalized. Unlike Swedish massage, in which the therapists apply their strokes to move blood toward the heart, Oriental massage therapists focus their work away from the heart to release blocked energy. (See Appendix A for information on how to find a certified Oriental massage practitioner.)

Oriental Massage for Diabetes

With your physician's consent, a full-body Oriental massage done by a professional is recommended. During a typical session, Oriental massage therapists often incorporate many different massage techniques, depending on whether the practitioner is performing *amma* or *tui ni,* and your particular needs.

A sample self-massage is presented here. It is part of a longer session that comes from the Anhui Medical School in China and is used by the Chinese to strengthen the body and prevent disease. Oriental massage practitioners emphasize that although the full series consists of twenty massage methods, you can select as many or as few as fits your particular circumstances. Practice this self-massage upon rising in the morning or before retiring at night.

Choose a quiet place where you won't be disturbed for about ten to fifteen minutes and sit in a comfortable chair.

• Rub your palms together thirty to forty times, increasing speed, until they are warm.

• Use your warmed hands to rub your face. Rub from the left side of the face across your forehead to the right side. Repeat this seven to eight times.

• Using the knuckles of your index, middle, and ring fingers of both hands, knead with a circular motion around your eye sockets. Begin at the inside corner and move to the outside, then go from the outside corner to the inside. Repeat seven to eight times each direction.

• Take the middle fingers of both hands and find the indentation just to the side of your eyes. Knead these points by making circles away from and then toward the eyes.

• With the tips of both middle fingers, make a wiping motion beginning from above and between your eyebrows outward to the points just to the side of your eyes.

• Place your palms at the hairline on the side of your head, directly above your ears and with your fingers pointing up. Using your palms, press firmly on both sides of your head at the hairline above your ears, then press on the front and back hairlines. Repeat on the sides and front and back thirty to forty times.

• Vibrate your ears by placing the fingers of both hands against the back of your head. Cover the ear canals with your palms and make a rapid, rhythmic drumming motion about thirty to forty times.

• Pat your chest by spreading the fingers of both hands and tapping against your chest with the flats of your fingers. Inhale with each tap. Repeat this seven to eight times.

• Use the outside edges of both hands to "chafe" (move rapidly in a sawlike motion) the two sides of your rib cage below your armpits. Do it quickly about thirty to forty times.

• Knead your abdomen by using your left palm to press on your umbilical area. Use your right hand to press on the back of the left. Apply as much pressure as is comfortable and knead your abdomen deeply in a clockwise direction thirty to eighty times.

• Massage your lower back by making fists with your hands, thumbs out, and quickly chafing both sides of your lower back thirty to forty times.

• To rub-roll your thighs, rest your legs in a bent position, feet flat on the floor. Place your palms on either side of one thigh and rub back and forth (left to right and vice versa). Move up and down the thigh. Rub-roll each thigh about thirty to forty times.

• Use the outside edge of your hand to chafe the spot that corresponds to the KD 1 (see Figure II-1) in acupressure. Chafe each foot thirty to forty times.

• Finish with a breath exercise. Stand with your legs shoulder width apart and hands at abdomen height, palms toward you. Lift your hands toward your throat and simultaneously lift your head, bend backward at the waist, and breathe in. Then lower your hands back to your abdomen, lower your head, bend forward at the waist, and breathe out. As you exhale, make the sounds "ha-ho-hee-hoo." Repeat this breath exercise twice.

In this age of highly technical medicine, many of the ancient healing practices not only continue to be used but are enjoying a resurgence. Oriental massage is being taught and practiced more and more in the West because it brings results for many people.

Swedish Massage

Swedish massage is probably the form most practiced in the United States, and it is used as the foundation for many other kinds of massage. It can offer you and other people with diabetes several therapeutic benefits, most notably its ability to induce the relaxation response (see Chapter 4 and the following pages). It also improves circulation, which helps prevent the circulatory problems associated with diabetes, and stimulates the functioning of the lymphatic system, which in turn controls the immune system. Swedish massage can even help with your exercise program by giving you more flexibility and range of motion.

How Does Swedish Massage Work?

As your muscles are massaged, several "switches" are turned on throughout your body. Massage sets the relaxation response into motion, which allows you to keep stress under control and, in turn, moderate your blood glucose levels. Other switches release neurochemicals called endorphins and enkephalins into your bloodstream. These chemicals are commonly referred to as "natural opiates," because they reduce or eliminate pain. Therefore Swedish massage may be helpful in relieving the pain associated with diabetic neuropathy.

The continuous pressure applied throughout a massage session causes an increase in blood and lymph circulation. Improved blood flow helps nutrients reach cells more efficiently and also removes toxins from your body faster. A more efficient lymph system, which is your body's primary defense against infection, is another benefit of massage.

Massage also has emotional benefits. Dealing with the everyday stress of having a chronic disease can be emotionally draining. Many people with diabetes have occasional or frequent bouts of depression. Massage satisfies a person's need for support and nurturing, promotes well-being, and reduces anxiety.

Swedish Massage for Diabetes

Swedish massage is not a do-it-yourself therapy, as it involves long, deep strokes, called *effleurage,* that provide the most benefit when you are the relaxed recipient. It is, however, an excellent healing art to learn and share with a spouse or friend. We recommend that you find a professional Swedish massage therapist or organization that can provide you and a partner with instructions, or visit a professional therapist for a complete treatment (see Appendix A).

The instructions below are merely a brief introduction to Swedish massage. They are for the back only, which is where Swedish massage usually begins, and are written for the person giving you the massage. Have the permission of your physician before receiving a massage.

If you do not have access to a massage table, make yourself comfortable on the floor using towels, blankets, a futon, sleeping bag, or a thin foam mattress. Place a pillow or a rolled-up towel under your knees, head, or neck when you lie faceup or under your ankles, pelvis, or chest when you lie facedown. For the massage explained below, you will lie facedown. Choose a location that allows your partner to kneel or stand comfortably above your head and on either side and to lean into muscles that need massage. If you choose to use baby oil or an herbal massage oil, you may want to warm it first.

Position yourself above the recipient's head so that when you look down the back of the recipient's head is directly below your face. If using oil, apply it to your palms and then, starting at the neck, slide your hands, palms down, along both sides of the spine along the length of the torso to the lower back. This long, gliding stroke is called *effleurage* and helps increase circulation. Repeat this motion several times. DO NOT massage the spine.

If the recipient can accept a deeper stroke, place one of your hands on top of the other one and apply *effleurage* on one side of the back at a time.

Next, position yourself to one side of the recipient at about shoulder level. With one or both hands, use your thumb and finger to "lift up" muscles away from the bones in the shoulder and then squeeze and knead them. This technique is called *pétrissage.* Use this technique all along the back and shoulders. *Pétrissage* improves circulation and stimulates delivery of nutrients to the cells.

When you do *pétrissage* in the lower back region and the recipient is on the floor rather than on a massage table, sit beside the recipient with your legs straight in front of you to help relieve strain on your back.

Next, position yourself above the shoulders. Apply friction by using the thumbs or fingertips of both hands to apply deep, circular movement on either side of the spine. To do this, insert your thumbs or fingers in the indentations along the vertebrae of the recipient and press your thumbs away from the spine. Go down the entire length of the spine.

After you have applied friction along the entire spine, use the *effleurage* technique again as you did in the first step.

Now position yourself to one side of the recipient just above waist level and perform *tapotement.* This technique involves either cupping your hands into a C-shape or using your knuckles, fists, or the flat of your hands to strike the muscles on the back with a chopping motion. If the recipient wants the muscles to be stimulated, use *tapotement* for only a few seconds. If, however, the muscles are cramped, strained, or in spasm, perform *tapotement* for at least ten seconds.

Finish the back massage with **vibration.** Place either your fingers or palms on both sides of the spine and press down while you rapidly vibrate your hands. This stroke stimulates the activity of the glands and boosts circulation.

A full-body Swedish massage is the most beneficial for people with diabetes and can provide all the advantages previously mentioned. Always get the consent of your physician before getting a massage, especially if you have blood vessel or heart problems.

Meditation

In homes, offices, clinics, and other types of meeting places across the United States, people with chronic diseases such as diabetes, hypertension, cancer, and heart disease are getting together and sitting in silence. To an outsider it looks as if they are not doing anything, but they are: they are concentrating on how it feels as the air goes in and out of their body. They are practicing a type of meditation called **sitting meditation.**

Dr. Bernie Siegel, who has done much research and writing on meditation, defines it as "an active process of focusing the mind into a state of relaxed awareness." There are many ways to achieve this, and sitting meditation is just one. Regardless of the type of meditation you practice—and we will explain several types below—the goal is the same: to bring yourself into a restful trance state that strengthens your mind by freeing it from the noise and confusion that usually occupy it.

How Does Meditation Work?

When you meditate, your body enters a state of calm. On a physical level, this means many things. (See the box, p. 146) Studies by Drs. Deepak Chopra, Herbert Benson, Jon Kabat-Zinn, Bernie Siegel, and others have shown, for example, that meditation reduces or normalizes stress hormone levels in the blood and brings about the relaxation response, a state of being in which the mind becomes clear of thoughts and activity. The body responds to this "mind-clearing'' with lower blood glucose levels, a lower heart and breathing rate, reduced blood pressure, and less oxygen consumption. It is a state of restful awareness.

Once your mind is uncluttered, you can think more clearly. This gives you an opportunity to explore how you feel about yourself and the fact that you have diabetes. Meditation allows you to face your fears without the presence of other thoughts. On a spiritual level, meditation allows you to experience inner peace and a feeling of connectedness to everything around you.

Meditation: An Introduction

There are two basic approaches to meditation, concentrative and mindfulness, and each approach has many variations. You can sample the variations other people have developed or create your own. Before you explore any variations, it is best to understand the basics so you have a place from which to start.

The realm of **concentrative meditation** was studied in the 1970s by Drs. Herbert Benson and R. Keith Wallace, who proved that this meditation approach can decrease heart rate, breathing rate, and oxygen consumption, often after only a few weeks of practice. In concentrative meditation, you focus your attention on a repetitive sound, image, or action in order to quiet your thoughts and your mind and increase your awareness. Some popular examples of repetitive meditative focuses include your breathing, a flickering candle flame, or a mantra. Repetitive meditative focuses are explained on pages 149–51, ''Choosing a Meditative Focus.''

Joan Borysenko, Ph.D., author of *Minding the Body, Mending the Mind* and *The Power of the Mind to Heal,* explains the concept of **mindfulness** succinctly when she says that it ''involves opening the attention to become aware of the continuously passing parade of sensations and feelings . . . without becoming involved in thinking about them.'' You are not alone if you feel this is nearly impossible to do. How do you ''not think''? Thoughts do creep into the mind, even of people who are adept at mindfulness meditation. Dr. Benson suggests adopting an oh-well attitude about infiltrating thoughts and just let them go. Such thoughts do serve an important purpose, however. Each time your thoughts intrude and you return to concentration, you strengthen your ''mental muscles of awareness and choice,'' says Borysenko. This commingling of physical and mental activity suggests that meditation is both a mental and a physical exercise. This connection is also demonstrated by the fact that when you stop meditation, the physical benefits usually disappear within a few weeks, as do any strength and endurance that are gained during physical exercise when you stop exercising.

MEDITATION POSE FOR YOGA

- Sit with your legs straight out in front of you and form a V shape.
- Bend your right leg and bring it toward you. Place your right foot on the floor close to your groin.
- Bend your left leg and place your left foot on the floor close to your right leg.
- Rest your hands on your knees: arms outstretched and palms up.
- Keep your back straight.

Meditation for Diabetes

Below are two meditations for you to try. The first is an example of concentrative meditation; the second, of mindfulness. Both can be used to help reduce tension, stress, and blood glucose levels. Some people find it helpful to tape meditations they find in books so they can just pop a cassette into their recorder and play the meditation of their choice. You also can purchase prerecorded meditations (see Appendix B).

CONCENTRATIVE MEDITATION

1. Choose the meditation pose for yoga previously described. Or:

2. Sit in a comfortable chair with your spine held straight and your eyes closed. Relax your shoulders, lift your chest, and let your chin fall lightly toward your throat. Place your hands on your knees, palms up. If you choose, connect the tips of your thumb and index finger of each hand.

3. Inhale deeply through your nose and slowly exhale. At the end of each exhalation, squeeze your buttocks and hold this position for a few seconds. Continue deep breathing and squeezing for about two minutes. Concentrate only on your breath and the squeeze.

4. After two minutes, switch your focus to any site that feels tense, tight, or painful. Perhaps you have a tension headache or your stomach is upset. Meditate on the spot that is causing you discomfort and breathe deeply into it. See that spot clearly in your mind. Continue to meditate on that spot and breathe deeply for about two minutes.

MINDFULNESS MEDITATION

1. Lie down flat on the floor or on a bed in a comfortable position. Place pillows under your head, knees, or lower back if needed.

2. Stretch slowly so you feel fully present in your body. Starting with your toes, do a brief inventory of your body parts as you stretch. Acknowledge each part's presence in your mind as you move from your toes to the top of your head.

3. Allow your eyes to close; take a deep breath and then exhale slowly and fully.

4. With your next breath, focus your attention to a spot just below your navel. Concentrate on sending each breath to that spot and be aware as it leaves, slowly and gently. Allow yourself to be fully aware of each breath as it enters that spot and leaves.

5. Now allow yourself to shift your attention away from that spot and become aware of your body. Focus on a spot that has pain, tension, or other distress. Perhaps your neck or shoulder muscles are tense; maybe you have a tension headache or are experiencing stomach discomfort. If you have more than one area that needs attention, focus on one at a time and finish with it completely before you move on to another spot. Imagine that you can send your breath to that spot. As you inhale, be aware of any sensations in the attention area. You can do this without judging whether these sensations are good or bad . . . they simply are.

6. As you exhale, notice if the feelings change. Let each breath wash over the area on which you have focused your attention. Acknowledge any sensations that arise and let them just be. Continue breathing in and out and acknowledging any sensations you are experiencing.

7. When you feel some relief at that spot, shift your focus to another spot that needs attention and repeat the process. Once you are ready to return to full consciousness, open your eyes and take a slow, deep breath and release it slowly.

With mindful meditation, do not be surprised if the tension or discomfort you focus on intensified at first. That's because you are sending your full attention to it. As you continue to meditate, however, the discomfort usually shifts, decreases, or even disappears. Do not get discouraged if you do not notice a significant difference the first few times you meditate. With practice, you can enjoy less stressful days and, hopefully, better control of your diabetes.

BENEFITS OF MEDITATION

- Induces the relaxation response.
- Can reduce blood glucose levels in people with high levels of stress.
- Increases alpha brain wave activity—the brain waves present during deep relaxation and creativity.
- Decreases the levels of stress hormones in the bloodstream.
- Reduces or normalizes blood pressure. In fact, meditation is recommended as the first line of therapy for mild cases of hypertension.
- Reduces pulse rate.
- Improves immune system resistance.
- Reduces lactate levels in the blood (lactate is related to high levels of anxiety).
- Evidence is that over time, it can increase memory, intelligence, creativity, and concentration.

Choosing a Meditative Focus

Here are some suggested meditative focuses. You may, of course, choose your own. One popular focus is the *mantra* or sound meditation, in which you use a word, syllable, or short phrase to help induce or deepen your concentration. Choose something that has special meaning for you and creates a sense of peace and security. *Love, peace, I am light,* and *joy* are some likely choices. Some people repeat parts of a prayer or use a syllable like *Om.*

A simple breath mantra involves slowly taking a single deep breath and saying the word *in* to yourself as you inhale and *out* as you exhale. After that single deep breath, do not try to control your breathing. Every time you inhale and exhale say the word *in* or *out* to yourself. Concentrate solely on repeating the words. Repeat your mantra aloud to yourself, saying it more and more softly until it is a whisper. Listen to it in your mind. You can close your eyes or keep them open, whatever is comfortable for you. You can speed up your mantra, make it get louder or softer, raise or lower the pitch. It doesn't matter; it is your mantra. Draw out the mantra so it takes up all your meditation: "innnnn" and "ouuuuuu-t." If your mind wanders, that's okay. Simply return to your words. Meditate for fifteen or twenty minutes or whatever is comfortable for you. When you are ready to return to full consciousness, do so gently. Take several slow, deep breaths and get up slowly.

Another technique is to focus on an object or place, real or imagined. You might choose a simple natural object: a tree, rock, flower, or acorn. You can even choose a space three to six feet ahead of you or a space on the other side of a wall. If you choose a real object, place it three or four feet in front of you at or near eye level. Sit comfortably and allow your eyes to rest on the object. Do not force your eyes to focus or not focus on the object—just rest your gaze upon it easily. When your eyes wander, which they will do, let them return to the object gently. Allow the object to remain in your field of vision for a comfortable amount of time—five to ten seconds for most people—and then let your eyes wander. Return your attention to the object whenever you are ready; you will "know" when the time is right for you. Every time you rest your eyes on the object, allow yourself to look at it innocently for five or ten seconds and then let your eyes wander again. Continue this for about five minutes. Then close your eyes for a moment and sit quietly.

People who practice daily meditation report feeling more rested and relaxed and better able to control shifts in blood glucose levels. Meditation helps them cope with stress during the day and thus gives them more confidence about their ability to control their diabetes. We recommend you make meditation a regular part of your daily routine. As little as fifteen or twenty minutes in the morning when you first get up or at night when you get home from work or school can be sufficient. You may find, however, that you want to do it longer: an hour of meditation each night, instead of watching television, may be the answer to bring down your stress level—and blood glucose level—at the end of a tension-filled day. For more information on meditation techniques, see the Bibliography and Suggested Readings.

Movement Therapy

Exercise has an image problem. It sounds like work and doesn't bring pictures of fun to mind. *Movement therapy* conjures up a more positive image. And a positive image of movement therapy is essential for you and everyone with diabetes, because exercise is a critical element in your management program.

Yet people with diabetes are not getting the exercise they need. Results of a recent study find that people with and without diabetes exercise about the same amount, and neither group is meeting national physical activity goals. Reasons for not exercising abound. People we spoke to blamed "time": no time, not enough time; they leave the house too early, get home too late. Some said they were too tired to exercise; others said it was too boring or they would if they had someone to exercise with them. We addressed all of

these excuses in Chapter 3. Now you have no excuses left
. . . so let's do it!

In this section we first discuss the ways movement therapy can help you control your diabetes and its associated complications. Then we look at several movement options and how they can benefit you. We hope we can encourage you to beat the statistics and move . . . while having fun!

How Does Movement Therapy Work?

Movement therapy is a type of "wonder drug" because it can provide so many benefits—and all without the high cost of medication. For people with diabetes, the list is impressive:

- Improves sensitivity to insulin, which means lower blood glucose levels and a reduced need for diabetes medication.
- Improves cardiovascular functioning (stronger, more efficient blood vessels and heart; improves blood circulation) and reduces risk of death from heart disease.
- Lowers total cholesterol and triglyceride levels (high levels are risk factors for heart disease).
- Reduces existing high blood pressure and reduces risk of developing high blood pressure.
- Increases strength and endurance.
- Reduces body fat and is key in weight loss and control.
- Reduces the risk of osteoporosis.
- Improves overall energy level and self-esteem.
- Reduces stress and muscle tension.

Exercise has a somewhat different effect on Type I and Type II diabetes. For people with Type I disease, exercise can help reduce the amount of insulin needed to keep blood glucose levels under control, but it cannot eliminate the requirement for insulin. In Type II diabetes, the majority of people are obese, and here movement therapy definitely can significantly reduce or eliminate their need for insulin or hypoglycemic pills, as well as prevent the need for either intervention.

Exercise increases the metabolism in the muscles. All it takes to raise your metabolism rate is twenty to thirty minutes of aerobic exercise. This increased metabolism rate can continue for many hours after you finish exercising. After strenuous exercise, for example, you may lower your blood glucose level for up to thirty-six hours.

Movement Therapy for Diabetes

Regular aerobic exercise is the cornerstone of a movement therapy plan for people with diabetes, especially Type II. Walking, jogging, swimming, rowing, aerobic dance, biking, cross-country skiing, handball, Rollerblading, ice skating, jumping rope, and using gym equipment such as a stair machine or rowing machine are all forms of aerobic movement. Before you dash out the door for a jog or dive into the pool, read the general guidelines for movement therapy.

• If your blood glucose level is less than 100 mg/dL before you plan to exercise, eat a snack containing about ten to twenty grams of carbohydrate. Some examples: half a bagel, one small apple or banana, four ounces of fruit juice, or three graham cracker squares.

• Do a warm-up and stretching for five to ten minutes before beginning the aerobic portion of your session. If you have chosen brisk walking as your movement, spend this time doing overall stretches and leg stretches and then walk at a normal pace.

• Spend at least twenty to thirty minutes doing an aerobic activity. If walking, gradually increase your pace and peak at about halfway through your allotted time. Take your pulse and see if you are under or over your target heart rate (see Table II-1, pp. 155–56). Adjust your walking speed to allow your heart rate to fall in your target area.

• End your session with a five- to ten-minute cooldown period of slow walking. At the end, do some overall and leg stretches.

If you take insulin, consider the following guidelines when exercising:

• Test your blood glucose level before and after exercise.

• The longer you exercise and/or the greater its intensity, the greater will be the drop in blood glucose level.

• Occasionally, a strenuous workout may cause blood glucose levels to rise because the liver releases more glucose than the muscles need. This possibility makes monitoring essential.

• If your exercise session lasts more than forty-five to sixty minutes, monitor your blood glucose level every hour and eat about fifteen grams of carbohydrate, if needed. If you plan on an entire day of activity, such as hiking or skiing, go prepared to monitor yourself and refuel as needed.

• Always carry quick-acting carbohydrate snacks with you (raisins, glucose tablets, hard candy, orange juice).

• If possible, keep your movement sessions on a consistent schedule; say, thirty minutes every morning before work or forty-five minutes after leaving work.

• Avoid injecting insulin into the muscles you will be exercising. There have been reports that exercising a limb within one to two hours of injection causes the insulin to act faster.

Moving into Your Program

We've given you movement therapy ideas and the guidelines. Now you just need to get started. If you haven't exercised in a while, you need to begin your movement therapy program slowly. You might begin with about ten to fifteen minutes of walking or riding a stationary bike. Over the next few weeks, gradually add a minute or so a day until you reach thirty to forty-five minutes for each session. Table II-1 shows you activity levels and suggested movement-therapy durations. It also shows you the target heart rate you should strive for during movement therapy. How do you know what your optimal heart rate should be during exercise? If you don't have high blood pressure, diabetic complications, or heart disease, use the formula below to figure your best rate. If you do have any of these conditions, consult with your physician or exercise physiologist.

TABLE II-1
YOU: ON THE MOVE!

If You Are:	Sessions Per Week	Minutes/ Session	Minutes/ Week	Heart Rate During Exercise
Sedentary	4–6	10–20	40–80	100–120
Slightly Active	4–6	15–30	90–120	100–130
Moderately Active	3–5	30–45	120–180	110–140
Very Active	3–5	30–60	180–300	120–160
Athletic	5–7	60–120	300–840	140–190

Consult your physician before beginning a movement therapy program. If you haven't been active for a while, begin with the sedentary guidelines.

Adapted from *The Joslin Guide to Diabetes*, 1995.

• Subtract your age from the number 220 (for example, if you are 40 years old, 40 from 220 is 180).

• To determine the heartbeat range you want to achieve during exercise, take 60 percent of 180 ($0.60 \times 180 = 108$) and 85 percent of 180 ($0.85 \times 180 = 153$).

• A healthy heart rate for you to achieve during movement therapy is 108 to 153 beats per minute.

• To check your heart rate while exercising, place the tip of a finger on your pulse on the thumb side of your wrist or on the side of your neck. Count the beats for ten seconds and then multiply that number by six.

Nutrition

Diabetes is associated intimately with food, thus attention to your diet is crucial for good control and management of the disease. The beauty of a diabetic eating plan is that it's not about eating differently; it's about eating smarter and healthier. Recommended eating plans for people with diabetes help maintain appropriate levels of blood glucose, cholesterol, and blood pressure as well as maintain a healthy weight—all goals that are good for both diabetics and nondiabetics alike.

In this section we explain how modifying your eating habits can have a significant impact on how well you manage your blood glucose levels and other aspects of diabetes. We then introduce several eating plans for diabetes. First are two approaches developed by physicians: the highly praised McDougall Program developed by Dr. John Mc-Dougall; and Gerson Therapy, established by Dr. Max Gerson. Both of these plans differ from the American Diabetes Association (ADA) traditional "food exchange" list, which is included here. We also have provided information about two variations of the ADA's food exchange list: the carbohydrate-counting plan and the fat-gram plan.

We urge you to find a physician or other diabetes health professional who is willing to explore dietary options and eating plans with you. Together you can create a plan that best suits you and your unique needs and lifestyle.

How a Healthy Food Plan Can Change Your Life

If you have Type II diabetes and are taking insulin or oral hypoglycemic medication, there is an excellent chance you can eliminate your need for these drugs if you change your diet. Up to 80 percent of people with Type II diabetes can stop taking insulin or oral diabetic medication and control their disease with diet and exercise alone. The remaining 20 percent can significantly reduce their need for medication. If you have Type I diabetes, you may be able to reduce your insulin intake by about one third when you follow a sound eating plan, such as one of those explained on the following pages.

If you are overweight, a healthy eating plan can help you shed those extra pounds, which will allow your body to make better use of insulin. A drop in weight will also reduce your risk of complications from diabetes, such as hypertension, heart disease, and stroke. When combined with movement therapy, a healthy eating plan will allow you to lose even more weight, as well as make you feel more vitality and energy.

General Dietary Considerations

The following guidelines were compiled from various sources involved in the management of diabetes and represent the wisdom from several successful food plans for diabetes.

• Eat five to six small meals a day: breakfast, lunch, and dinner, with a snack between each meal and then a nighttime snack if desired or needed. This helps maintain a steady blood sugar level.

• Reduce salt intake: it reduces blood glucose levels. Avoid foods that have a high salt content, such as pickled foods, olives, snack foods, frozen dinners, canned soups and other canned items, and fast foods. Learn to use various herbs and spices instead. You also can use seaweeds, which have a salty flavor.

• Consumption of meat can cause sugar cravings in your body's attempt to establish a protein/carbohydrate balance. Excessive meat consumption also produces prostaglandins that cause pain, inflammation, and depression. It is best to avoid meat and meat products.

• Avoid foods containing sugar, honey, glucose, glucose syrup, dextrose, and fructose: candy, cakes, cookies, puddings, sweetened cereals, and condiments such as ketchup and barbecue sauce. As substitutes, use sugarcane molasses for sweetening in cooking; instead of honey, use unsweetened jam.

• Foods high in fiber, especially soluble fiber, should be a central part of your diet. Soluble fiber, found in vegetables, oats, and fruit, increases the time it takes for the intestines to absorb glucose and help maintain optimal blood glucose levels.

• Avoid refined and processed foods. Whole, natural foods are used by the body more slowly and evenly, which allows better maintenance of blood glucose levels.

• High-protein diets are dangerous, especially for people with diabetes. Excessive protein, especially animal protein, causes the kidneys to work overtime and excrete large amounts of calcium from the body. The result can be kidney disease and osteoporosis.

• Avoid alcohol, as it can impair how your body handles sugar

• Avoid soft water. Diabetes is higher in soft water areas.

Drink natural, noncarbonated mineral or spring water that contains naturally occurring trace minerals. Clinical studies have shown that a good supply of trace minerals is important for effective glucose tolerance and utilization.

• You *deserve* good, healthy food. Create time in your schedule to shop for fresh fruits and vegetables. Eat at home more often, learn how to use a steamer, and don't fry foods. Take a diabetic cooking class or cook with a friend. Make it FUN.

• Don't let yourself get hungry, because you'll have a tendency to reach for something quick—and unhealthy. Keep dried fruit, whole grain crackers, or popcorn with you to snack on.

AMERICAN DIABETES ASSOCIATION NUTRITIONAL GUIDELINES

The American Diabetes Association (ADA) has established the following nutritional recommendations for people with diabetes. An increasing number of physicians, however, believe these guidelines are inappropriate. Two food plans that reflect that opinion are included in this section: the McDougall Program and Gerson Therapy. Others, including the work of Julian M. Whitaker, M.D. (founder of the Whitaker Wellness Institute and author of *Reversing Diabetes*) and Nathan Pritikin, M.D., founder of Nathan Pritikin's Longevity Center, are not discussed here but are recommended reading. See the Suggested Reading List.

• Carbohydrates: Although the percentage of calories people with diabetes should get from carbohydrates depends on their individual needs and management goals, the ADA's recommended range is 60 to 65 percent of calories from carbohydrates.

• Protein: If you do not have signs of kidney disease, the

ADA recommends between 10 and 20 percent of calories be derived from protein. Many physicians recommend the lower end of the range as a precaution against kidney problems. If you already have kidney disease, protein intake should be limited to about forty-three grams if you weigh 120 pounds, fifty-four grams if 150 pounds, and sixty-five grams if 180 pounds.

• Fat: Here the range is 10 to 30 percent, with no more than 10 percent of calories coming from saturated fat. Saturated fat comes primarily from animal products (meat, dairy foods) and a few plant sources such as coconut and palm oil. Your remaining fat intake should come from unsaturated or polyunsaturated fats, such as safflower, sunflower, corn, or soybean oils; or from monounsaturated fats, found in olive and canola oil, peanuts, and most nuts and seeds.

• Cholesterol: Less than 300 milligrams per day.

• Fiber: The recommended intake of twenty-five to thirty grams per day is the same as for the general population. The ADA recommends that fiber should come from your food and not from fiber supplements.

• Sodium: No more than 2,400 to 3,000 milligrams per day. If you have mild to moderate high blood pressure, 2,400 milligrams or less per day is recommended.

The McDougall Program

The McDougall Program is a high-fiber, high-carbohydrate, ultra–low-fat, no-cholesterol, starch-based food program that is being used successfully for treatment of diabetes, heart disease, and hypertension. (Exercise is also part of the program but is not discussed in this Nutrition segment.) It was developed by John McDougall, M.D., best-selling author and medical director of the McDougall Program at St. Helena Hospital in Deer Park, California.

Individuals who adopt this program report significant results: Type I diabetics typically reduce their insulin requirements by 30 percent and their blood glucose levels become more stable. For those with Type II diabetes, the program allows 75 percent of patients to stop taking all insulin, and more than 95 percent stop taking all hypoglycemic pills.

An added benefit for individuals in both groups is a reduction in the risk of complications. Many of the complications that occur with diabetes are the result of eating a rich diet, which burdens the diabetic's weakened system. In the United States, even mild changes in blood glucose control are associated with an increased rate of heart attack. In countries where the people eat a starch-based diet, however, atherosclerosis is uncommon among the few cases of diabetes that do occur.

How the McDougall Plan Works

"Instead of the diet high in fats, protein, and refined foods . . . switch to a low-fat diet offering much more carbohydrates and fiber," says Dr. McDougall in *McDougall's Medicine.* "The proportions for this ideal diet are 80 to 90 percent carbohydrates, 5 to 12 percent protein, and 5 to 10 percent fats, with no cholesterol at all, and a high content of fiber. This kind of diet will reduce the blood sugar levels of most diabetics (both types)." You can follow McDougall's program, either on your own (with your management team's guidance, naturally; see *McDougall's Medicine* in the Bibliography and Suggested Reading), or at St. Helena's, which offers a twelve-day program to get people started. During the initial twelve days on the McDougall Program, the average drop in cholesterol is nearly 28 mg/dL, with many people achieving a 100 mg/dL drop without taking hypertension drugs. The average drop in cholesterol for the same time period is 67 mg/dL for those who start the program with levels higher than 300 mg/dL, and 23 to

37 mg/dL for those with a beginning cholesterol of 200 to 299 mg/dL. Individuals who are overweight when they begin the program lose an average of six to fifteen pounds of fat per month while consuming completely balanced, high-carbohydrate, satisfying meals.

THE MCDOUGALL PROGRAM FOR DIABETES

For people with Type II diabetes who enter the program at St. Helene's, those taking diabetes pills are taken off their medication immediately by Dr. McDougall, while those on insulin reduce their dosage by at least one half. This is the same approach he recommends for those who use the program under the supervision of their management team. Blood glucose levels need to be monitored closely, as the switch to the new eating plan causes significant changes in sugar levels. Hypoglycemic events are possible during this initial phase, so always have fruit juice or hard candy readily available. For individuals with Type I diabetes, Dr. McDougall reduces their insulin dosages by 30 percent when they enter the program and make additional adjustments as needed. Generally, for people with either Type I or Type II diabetes, Dr. McDougall recommends keeping blood glucose levels slightly high rather than low during this transition period to avoid hypoglycemic episodes.

Basically, the McDougall Program includes starchy (for example, corn, potatoes) and all other vegetables, whole grains, pastas, beans, legumes, fruits, soy products, seeds, and nuts (the last three in limited quantities after the initial twelve days). Salt-free and low-sodium seasonings are encouraged, and table sugar should be replaced by honey, pure maple syrup, or no-sugar pure fruit spreads. The program includes a list of "free foods" and snacks that can be eaten in unlimited amounts. For a complete food list, as well as menu plans and recipes, see *The McDougall Program: Twelve Days to Dynamic Health, McDougall's Medi-*

cine: A Challenging Second Opinion, and *The McDougall Health-Supporting Cookbook* (see the Bibliography and Suggested Reading). A few sample menu plans are reproduced below.

BREAKFAST: Fresh fruit or fruit juice
"Fried" potatoes
Herbal tea

LUNCH: Garbanzo bean soup
Tomatoes with salsa
Whole wheat bread or pita bread
Fresh fruit
Soda water

DINNER: Cajun rice
Tossed green salad with oil-free dressing
Frozen fruit dessert
Hot or cold herbal tea

BREAKFAST: Fresh fruit or fruit juice
Hot breakfast quinoa
Herbal tea

LUNCH: Pita bread stuffed with beans and vegetables
Fresh fruit
Soda water

DINNER: Pasta primavera
Cauliflower
Fruit pudding
Hot or cold herbal tea

The McDougall Program is not a diet: it is a way of eating for the rest of your life. It was developed to be diversified, filling, and nutritious so people would find it easy and convenient to follow. If you would like to reduce or eliminate your dependence on diabetes medications, lose weight, and achieve better overall health, the McDougall Program may be for you.

Gerson Therapy

Gerson Therapy is an intensive nutrition therapy that works closely with nature and is based on the idea that simple foods, juices, and nontoxic medications can help rid the body of disease. It was developed by Dr. Max Gerson, a German-born physician whose search to cure his own medical problems led him to discover the healing powers of clean (organically grown) fruits, vegetables, and grains, ultra–low-fat intake, and high intake of nutrients in treating diabetes, tuberculosis, and cancer. In the 1950s, Dr. Gerson wrote that a diet consisting of 75 percent nutritious foods outlined in the Gerson Therapy plan and 25 percent of an individual's choice was adequate for good health. Today, however, increased pollution of the water and air, the burgeoning use of chemicals in foods and in the soil, and the depletion of nutrients in the soil have caused the Gerson Institute to recommend these figures be changed to 90 percent and 10 percent in order to prevent disease. For individuals with diabetes, 100 percent is optimum.

People who want to adopt Gerson Therapy need to work with an individual trained in Gerson Therapy to develop an eating plan that is specific for them. See Appendix A for information on how to contact the Gerson Institute.

How Gerson Therapy Works

According to the Gerson Institute, Gerson Therapy helps prevent Type II diabetes because it is a low–animal protein, low-fat, low-salt diet that focuses on optimizing the body's immune system and high enzyme functioning. Gerson Therapy program is based on the fact that in individuals with Type II diabetes, the insulin receptors on the body's cells are blocked or clogged with cholesterol and prevent the insulin from entering and thus allowing glucose to penetrate the cell membrane. Gerson Therapy eliminates cholesterol from and greatly reduces fat in the diet, which in turn allows an individual's own insulin to move freely in the body. This approach also allows the body to break down and eliminate arteriosclerosis, the risk of kidney and eye problems, as well as stress on the heart. Gerson Therapy also provides optimal nutrition and helps the body to detoxify. By ridding the body of toxins, all the body systems can be restored to health. In people with diabetes, metabolism is normalized and the body can heal itself.

When people first adopt Gerson Therapy, their blood glucose levels are monitored constantly so their insulin or pills can be withdrawn safely. Charlotte Gerson, president of the Gerson Institute, explains that people with diabetes who choose Gerson Therapy often experience a dramatic drop in blood cholesterol levels in as little as one week. Some see a reduction as high as 100 points, and without using cholesterol-reducing drugs. Along with this reduction in cholesterol also comes a decrease in requirements for insulin supplementation. For people with Type I diabetes, Gerson Therapy can help improve eyesight and overcome high blood pressure and kidney damage when the diet is followed faithfully.

THE GERSON EATING PLAN

The eating plan is based on several features, including:

- Consumption of fresh, raw, organic fruits and vegetables and organic grains
- Restricted salt intake
- Potassium supplements
- Ultra–low-fat intake
- Occasional (temporary) restriction of protein intake
- High intake of vitamins, minerals, and micronutrients

- Plenty of fluid intake
- Avoidance of alcohol, caffeine, drugs and other stimulants, and fried foods

Advocates of Gerson Therapy believe that consumption of specific raw fruits and vegetables and their juices supply much more nutritional benefits than scientists have been able to identify thus far. Therefore, people who follow Gerson Therapy drink thirteen glasses of various fresh raw juices daily, all of which are prepared from organically grown vegetables and fruits.

Gerson Therapy also involves use of biological medications, such as castor oil, pancreatic enzymes, and a liver extract with vitamin B_{12}, and enemas of coffee or chamomile tea. The addition of biological agents to the eating plan support optimal enzyme activity and functioning of the immune system. The enemas remove toxins from the tissues and blood by stimulating the enzyme systems in the stomach wall and liver and promote the elimination of toxic bile.

PREVENTING DIABETES WITH GERSON THERAPY

According to advocates of Gerson Therapy, Type I diabetes can be prevented, and that prevention begins with the mother. Even before a woman is pregnant, a diet high in fat, salt, and protein—the Standard American Diet (SAD)—is harmful to both the mother and the unconceived child. The recommended diet for before, during, and after pregnancy is one consisting primarily of fresh (organic if possible) vegetables and fruit, juices, raw salads, and a minute amount of nonfat, unsalted protein food such as nonfat soy yogurt or cottage cheese. Stimulants such as tobacco, coffee, alcohol, and any kind of doctor-prescribed or street drugs should be avoided. The Gerson Institute strongly disputes the claim that drinking lots of milk during pregnancy is beneficial; in fact, milk can overload the kidneys and lead to toxemia, disturbances to the metabolism that can cause problems during pregnancy and the birth.

After the birth, the Gerson approach emphasizes the importance of breast feeding, especially the transparent fluid, called **colostrum,** that first enters the breast. This fluid helps build the baby's immune system. Even before infants are ready for solid foods, Gerson Therapy recommends giving them freshly pressed organic carrot juice. When infants are ready for solid foods, Gerson advocates fresh, live foods such as vegetables, mashed bananas and apples, and oatmeal rather than processed foods.

The word from the Gerson Institute is that Gerson Therapy "is totally nonspecific; by correcting the nutrition and helping the body to detoxify, all the body systems can be reactivated and restored, the metabolism is normalized, and the body can heal itself of chronic/degenerative disease." Although some people find Gerson Therapy does not fit into their lifestyle, it is a healthy alternative to conventional diabetes eating plans.

Food Exchange Meal Plan

Both the American Diabetes Association and the American Dietetic Association joined forces to develop a food program that can help people with diabetes plan meals that contain the proper amount of protein, carbohydrate, fat, and calories for their specific needs and lifestyle and to maintain normal blood glucose levels. This program is based on six groups of foods called exchange lists: starch/bread, meat and meat substitutes, vegetables, fruit, milk/soy milk, and fat. In addition to these six groups, there are two other lists: "free foods," which have twenty calories or less per serving; and combination foods, items such as vegetable lasagna or chili, which consist of foods from several lists. Two variations of the Food Exchange Meal Plan—carbohydrate-gram counting and fat-gram counting—are also discussed below.

Ask your dietitian or diabetes educator for a complete list of the foods in the exchange lists. Or, contact your local American Diabetes Association or American Dietetics Association office or see the Bibliography and Suggested Reading at the end of this book for more information.

HOW AN EXCHANGE MEAL PLAN WORKS

You and your dietitian can work together to determine the number of choices you need from each food group for each meal that will best control your blood glucose levels. A "choice" is a predetermined amount of food that contains a set number of grams of protein, carbohydrate, fat, and calories. Because all the foods within any given group contain nearly the same amount of nutrients and calories, you can "exchange" one item for any other in the same group. Within "Fruit," for example, to fulfill your fruit requirement for lunch you could choose one-half grapefruit, one small apple, one cup of cantaloupe, or fifteen small grapes. All of these items contain fifteen grams of carbohydrates, zero grams protein, zero grams fat, and sixty calories.

A sample exchange meal plan is shown in Figure II-2. It shows a sample menu for an entire day. Your meal plan will differ and be based on the following factors:

YOUR NUTRIENT AND CALORIC NEEDS

Here you need to consider factors such as whether you need to lose some weight or if you have special nutrient needs because of pregnancy or a medical condition.

• Your lifestyle. Your meal plan needs to reflect your daily routine or you probably will not follow it. If you work nights or have a long commute to and from work or school, for example, you need to plan your meals and snacks at

MENU PLAN

NAME _____   DATE _____

DIETITIAN _____   PHONE _____

	Grams	Percent
Carbohydrate	_____	_____
Protein	_____	_____
Fat	_____	_____
Calories	_____	

TIME	MEAL PLAN	FOOD ITEMS/IDEAS
	——— Starch	
	——— Meat/Substitute	
	——— Vegetable	
	——— Fruit	
	——— Milk Substitute	
	——— Fat	
	———	
	———	
	——— Starch	
	——— Meat/Substitute	
	——— Vegetable	
	——— Fruit	
	——— Milk Substitute	
	——— Fat	
	———	
	———	
	——— Starch	
	——— Meat/Substitute	
	——— Vegetable	
	——— Fruit	
	——— Milk Substitute	
	——— Fat	
	———	
	———	
	———	

Fig. II-2

times that both fit your schedule and maintain normal blood glucose levels.

• How you control your diabetes. If you take insulin, you need to coordinate your food intake with your insulin injections. If you are taking hypoglycemic pills, you also need to match your meals and snacks with the action of your medication. Careful timing of meals is not as critical, however, if you control diabetes with diet alone, although spreading out your meals and snacks is recommended to help control blood glucose levels.

• Your activity level. This factor affects your daily caloric needs as well as the amount of medication and food you may need. If you take insulin, exercise can lower your blood glucose levels, which triggers the need for additional food to maintain those levels. If you manage your diabetes with diet alone, exercise helps your body control blood glucose levels.

Some people say the Food Exchange Meal Plan is too restrictive or cumbersome; others say they like knowing exactly what and how much they should eat. With the introduction of more meat and dairy substitutes on the market, people with diabetes who choose to eliminate animal foods from their diet find the Food Exchange Meal Plan easier to use. If this plan does not work for you, explore other options along with your dietitian or diabetes educator.

Carbohydrate Counting Plan

This approach to food planning became popular in 1994 when the American Diabetes Association announced that results of the DCCT indicated that it makes little difference whether people with diabetes eat ten grams of pasta or ten grams of white sugar: the effect on blood glucose levels is the same. This led to the introduction of a variation of the Food Exchange Plan: carbohydrate counting, which focuses on the total amount of carbohydrates you consume at a given meal or snack.

You and your dietitian still must determine your carbohydrate needs for each meal and snack, and then you can choose which foods will satisfy that amount. For example, if you should eat sixty grams of carbohydrates for dinner, you may choose one-third cup of lentils (fifteen grams), one-third cup of rice (fifteen grams), and a piece of angel food cake (thirty grams) to satisfy your sweet tooth. Or you could cut out the cake and add one cup of broccoli (ten grams), an ear of corn (fifteen grams), and one-half cup of tomato juice (five grams) to the lentils and rice.

Carbohydrate counting allows you more meal-planning flexibility and more food choices. It also provides you with a way to more precisely match your food selections with your activity level and medication, which can ultimately lead to better blood glucose control.

Fat-Gram Counting Plan

Fat-gram counting is another approach offered by the ADA. It involves counting fat grams instead of carbohydrate grams and can be a useful approach if you need to lose weight. By reducing the amount of fat in your diet, you can lose the fat that is interfering with the effectiveness of insulin in your body.

Your dietitian can determine how many fat grams you need to maintain good health and blood glucose control. Because every fat gram contains twice as many calories as carbohydrates and protein, this meal plan allows you to eat more high-carbohydrate foods. Another high-carbohydrate eating plan, which also is ultra–low fat and contains no cholesterol, is the McDougall Program, which is helpful for those who need to lose weight.

Nutritional Supplements

In addition to the foods in your eating plans, nutritional supplements can have a significant, positive effect on controlling blood glucose levels and in preventing some of the long-term complications of diabetes, such as heart disease, cataracts, retinopathy, and neuropathy. In this section, we look at some of the vitamins, minerals, and other nutrients that can provide you with these benefits. *Before you start any supplement program, consult with your physician and diabetes management team.* We also recommend that you consult with a naturopath. Unlike most physicians, naturopaths are trained in nutrition and supplementation (see Chapter 2).

Bioflavonoids

Bioflavonoids are antioxidants—substances that boost the immune system, among many other essential functions. They are found in highest concentrations in herbs and spices, including cayenne, thyme, turmeric, rosemary, garlic, and unfermented green tea. The primary functions of bioflavonoids are to strengthen blood vessel walls—which in turn helps prevent stroke, bruising, bleeding gums, and other blood vessel–related problems—improve insulin secretion, and prevent vitamin C from being destroyed. Bioflavonoid supplements are available individually, as a complex, or combined with vitamin C and other supplements. The average daily dose of quercetin and rutin (two of the most common bioflavonoids on the market) is two hundred to five hundred milligrams. If you buy a bioflavonoid complex, the average dose is five hundred to a thousand milligrams daily. As a preventive measure against diabetic complications, some experts recommend taking two thousand milligrams daily. Another important bioflavonoid is pycnogenol, which, when combined with vitamin C, increases the strength of capillary walls.

B Vitamins

Of the B vitamins, niacin (B_3), thiamine (B_1), pantothenic acid (B_5), pyridoxine (B_6), and B_{12} metabolize carbohydrates and fats, increase insulin's effectiveness, and help prevent symptoms of diabetes. People with diabetes who have deficiencies or imbalances of B vitamins often have trouble regulating their blood glucose levels. A general word of advice when taking B vitamins: Taking individual B vitamins can contribute to or cause an imbalance among other B vitamins in your body (as well as be costly and bothersome to take). Therefore, experts recommend taking a B vitamin complex that supplies the dosages prescribed by your management team, dietitian, or nutritionist.

Niacin is perhaps the most important B vitamin in terms of balancing blood glucose levels. *Niacin* is the term commonly used to refer to the two forms of vitamin B_3: nicotinic acid and nicotinamide. Niacin is an essential component of **glucose tolerance factor (GTF),** a nutrient that increases the ability of insulin to function properly (see "Chromium," p. 174). A niacin deficiency can hinder the body's ability to regulate blood glucose levels. According to Melvyn Werbach, M.D. (author of *Healing with Food*), even diabetics who have normal niacin levels can better regulate their blood glucose levels if they take niacin supplements. Because many people have a negative reaction to niacin (temporary flushing, tingling in the arms and legs, burning, and itching), take vitamin B_3 in the nicotinamide form. Check the label on your vitamin bottle.

The recommended daily supplement of B_3 is 50 to 100 milligrams. To help prevent diabetic kidney disease, Dr. Werbach suggests 650 milligrams of nicotinamide daily.

Thiamine (vitamin B_1) levels are low in many people

with diabetes. A severe deficiency can cause neuropathy (a disease of the nervous system), while supplements may improve sensory neuropathy. Research continues in this area. As a safeguard, Dr. Werbach recommends fifty milligrams of thiamine daily for diabetics with diabetic neuropathy.

Vitamin B_6 (pyridoxine) appears in low levels in many diabetics, yet the effectiveness of supplementation is still unknown. Some studies show that it can improve glucose tolerance in pregnant women who are vitamin B_6 deficient and who develop diabetes during pregnancy (gestational diabetes). Advocates of supplementing with vitamin B_6 say it can reduce symptoms of neuropathy or that it helps prevent complications in long-standing diabetes, while others claim it has no benefit (see the Bibliography and Suggested Reading). If you and your physician decide vitamin B_6 may help you, the suggested dosage is 50 mg twice daily.

Vitamin B_{12} injections given to people with diabetes have been effective in relieving neuropathy. Oral forms of this vitamin are ineffective for this purpose, however.

Biotin appears to enhance insulin's action and increase the activity of the enzyme glucokinase, which is responsible for the first step in the utilization of glucose in the liver. People with diabetes typically have low levels of biotin; to improve glucokinase activity and glucose metabolism, supplement with fifteen milligrams daily.

Chromium

Chromium is a trace element that plays a major role in glucose tolerance factor (GTF), a substance that is necessary for the proper function of insulin. Chromium works closely with insulin to help glucose be accepted into the cells. A deficiency of chromium blocks the ability of insulin to do its job, thus glucose levels rise. Some experts believe a chromium deficiency can cause Type II diabetes. Many people with diabetes who take chromium supplements have experienced improved glucose tolerance and better regulation of blood glucose levels, although others report no benefit. Some people with diabetes use chromium drops to help control sugar cravings. Yet according to the ADA's Nutrition Recommendations and Principles for People with Diabetes Mellitus, ''it appears that most people with diabetes are not chromium deficient and, therefore, chromium supplementation has no known benefit.'' Investigation into the role of chromium in diabetes continues.

If you and your management team decide you will take chromium, the average dose for adults is two hundred to six hundred micrograms per day. Chromium is available as tablets, capsules, and liquid and comes in various forms: as chromium polynicotinate, which contains chromium and niacin (which causes flushing and itching in some individuals); as chromium picolinate; and as a combination of chromium picolinate, GTF, and other nutrients. Another source of chromium is brewer's yeast, which contains a concentrated source of GTF as well. Brewer's yeast is available as flakes, powder, tablets, and capsules and in a wide range of potencies, so check the label. Generally, a tablespoon of dried brewer's yeast contains fifty to seventy milligrams of chromium.

Coenzyme Q

This natural substance, also known as Co-Q-10, is one of many coenzymes in the body that ''buddy up'' with enzymes to help them perform their specific functions. It is believed coenzyme Q works at a cellular level to improve the utilization of oxygen. Dr. Andrew Weil *(Spontaneous Healing; Natural Health, Natural Healing)* recommends that people with diabetes take eighty milligrams a day for three months to stabilize blood glucose levels.

Copper

Copper is an essential nutrient; however, do not take a supplement until your physician has determined that you have a deficiency. If you have abnormally low copper levels and you routinely eat sugar, a substance called sorbitol, a glucose derivative, can collect in your tissues and lead to the development of neuropathy, cataracts, retinopathy, and other diabetic complications. The suggested dosage of copper for deficiency is two to four milligrams daily.

Essential Fatty Acids

Omega-3 and omega-6 essential fatty acids are essential because the body needs them but cannot produce them. Of the two, omega-6, which consists of linoleic acid and its derivatives, appears to reduce the risk of microangiopathy (small blood vessel disease) and heart ischemia (inadequate blood flow from the coronary arteries) in people with diabetes. A good source of omega-6 is the oil of the evening primrose plant, which is also rich in gamma-linolenic acid (GLA), an oil that is obtained from linolenic acid. This oil reportedly can reverse nerve damage to peripheral nerves in patients with diabetic neuropathy. The recommended dosage for treatment of diabetic neuropathy is one gram four times daily.

GLA oils regulate insulin and seem to protect against diabetic heart, eye, and kidney damage. Omega-3 oils help cleanse the heart and arteries. Linoleic fatty acid has an insulin-sparing activity that allows insulin to be more effective. Fresh flax seed oil contains high-quality linoleic acid and omega-3 fatty acids. Omega-6 can be found in evening primrose, borage, and black currant seed oils (take enough of any concentrated form that supplies 150–350 milligrams of GLA daily) and spirulina. The 150-milligram dose is adequate for vegetarians who eat mostly unprocessed foods; higher doses are needed for individuals on other diets.

Fiber

Fiber is the part of plants that cannot be digested or absorbed by the body. It is a carbohydrate that is obtained from whole grains, vegetables, fruits, nuts, and seeds. Fiber is either water soluble (dissolves in water) or water insoluble (does not dissolve in water). Water-soluble fiber is especially good for people with diabetes because as it slows down the passage of food through your system, it helps control blood glucose levels, reduces cholesterol levels, and possibly decreases the need for insulin. Water-insoluble fiber helps move waste materials through your intestines.

It is best to get all the fiber you need through the food you eat, although fiber supplements can provide extra help in lowering cholesterol levels and helping control blood glucose levels. If you and your dietitian decide you need fiber supplements, add them slowly to your diet: four to five grams once per day to start, gradually increasing to two to three times per day as your body adjusts. It is essential to drink at least six to eight glasses of water per day to prevent fiber supplements from causing constipation.

Magnesium

This nutrient is involved in glucose metabolism. Magnesium deficiency is common among people with diabetes, and very low levels are common among people with severe retinopathy. Magnesium supplements may also help prevent complications of heart disease.

In addition to a diet rich in magnesium (see Table II-2, pp. 181–182), a supplement of three hundred to five hundred milligrams of magnesium daily is recommended for people with diabetes. Magnesium needs a "key" to get inside the cells of the body, and vitamin B_6 is that key. At least fifty milligrams per day of vitamin B_6 is recommended (see p. 174). For individuals with high blood pressure, a combination of five hundred to a thousand milligrams of magnesium and one thousand to fifteen hundred milligrams of calcium is recommended.

Manganese

Manganese serves an important role in glucose metabolism, which is of interest given that people with diabetes have only half the manganese of people without diabetes. Low manganese levels also have been suggested as a significant risk factor for the development of cardiovascular disease.

The suggested dosage of manganese for individuals with Type I diabetes is three to five milligrams daily. Because supplementation with manganese may change the insulin needs of people with Type I diabetes, careful monitoring is essential.

Phosphorus

A phosphorus deficiency can cause your body to respond abnormally to insulin, and supplementation may correct this problem. Phosphorus also may have a role in helping the red blood cells of people with Type I diabetes release oxygen to the tissues, a problem that occurs in this form of diabetes. Increasing the oxygen supply can help prevent diabetic angiopathy and increase energy levels. The suggested dosage of phosphorus is one gram three times daily with meals.

Vanadium

The FDA has not yet established an RDA for this trace element. Results of animal studies suggest that vanadium may help to control blood glucose fluctuations, although its effect in humans has not been determined. A daily supplemental dose of one hundred micrograms is considered safe; one milligram or more may be toxic. Vanadium comes in several forms. Recommended formulas include bis(maltolato)oxo vanadium complex (BMOV) and the vanadyl sulfate form.

Vitamin C

People with diabetes have abnormal vitamin C metabolism, which can result in low levels of the vitamin in the blood even when dietary intake is adequate. Vitamin C is especially important in people with Type I diabetes, as insulin facilitates the transport of vitamin C. Chronic low levels of vitamin C can lead to poor wound healing, an increased tendency to bleed, raised cholesterol levels, and a depressed immune system. Daily supplementation with one thousand to three thousand milligrams can help stabilize blood glucose levels in people with Type II diabetes, help prevent heart disease, and reduce small blood vessel fragility. Some experts recommend doses up to five thousand milligrams daily.

Vitamin E

Increased intake of this vitamin may help people with Type I diabetes reduce their insulin requirement. Under the guidance of your physician, start with no more than 100 IU of vitamin E daily and increase the dosage slowly. The recommended dose is 400 to 800 IU/day. Because selenium works closely with vitamin E, a supplement of two hundred to four hundred micrograms of selenium is recommended if you take high doses of vitamin E.

Vitamin E also appears to help prevent blood vessel disease. In people with diabetes, the platelets have a tendency to clump together, which can lead to blood vessel disease. Vitamin E helps prevent clumping and reduces the fat levels in the blood.

Zinc

Zinc plays a key role in the production and metabolism of insulin and helps prevent blood glucose imbalances. A zinc deficiency is believed to increase the risk of developing diabetes. The optimal daily dose of zinc, best taken in a multimineral supplement that contains copper, selenium, and iron, is seventeen to thirty milligrams, taken with food.

Zinc protects against beta cell destruction. Diabetics usually excrete too much zinc in the urine and so need supplementation. Zinc also is used to treat advanced hardening of the arteries.

FUN FOOD FACTS
FOODS THAT INCREASE THE ACTION
OF INSULIN

• Onions and garlic. Use these foods liberally. Make An onion a day your motto.

• Chromium-rich foods such as brewer's yeast, whole wheat bread, wheat bran, rye bread, and potatoes.

• Zinc-rich foods such as ginger root, wheat germ, pecans, brazil nuts, and split peas.

• Foods high in water-soluble fiber: flax seed, pectin, guar gum, oat bran, mucilage.

• Whole grain and legume carbohydrates, such as squash, sweet potatoes, and carrots.

• Pumpkin, whole rice, yams, mung beans, string beans, cucumber, celery, peach, millet, spinach, blueberry, peas, tofu, cabbage, daikon radish, mulberries.

• Foods rich in iodine, silicon, phosphorus such as kelp, Swiss chard, turnip greens, lecithin, sesame seed butter, seeds, and nuts.

> • Spices such as cinnamon, turmeric, bay leaf, and
> cloves, which are used in East India to control diabetes.

TABLE II-2
RDA VALUES AND FOOD SOURCES OF SELECTED NUTRIENTS

Nutrient	RDA	Food Sources
Magnesium	280–350 mg	Whole grains, leafy green vegetables, seeds, nuts, legumes
Zinc	10–15 mg/day	Soybeans, wheat bran, wheat germ, whole-grain foods, sesame and sunflower seeds
Chromium	50–200 mcg/day	Brewer's yeast, wheat germ, legumes, beans, peas, molasses
Vitamin B_6	10–15 mg/day	Wheat germ, whole grains, soybeans, dried beans, prunes, bananas, potatoes
Niacin	13–19 mg	Tofu, soybeans, bulgar wheat, peas, beans (mung, navy, lima, pinto, kidney), lentils
Vitamin C	60 mg	Citrus, papaya, tomatoes, guava, broccoli, cantaloupe, peppers, strawberries
Thiamine	1.5 mg	Brewer's yeast, whole wheat, pinto beans, peas, wheat germ, soybeans, barley, lima beans
Copper	1.5–3 mg	Avocados, bananas, potatoes, spinach, peas
Manganese	—	Whole-grain products
Vitamin E	30 IU	Almonds, walnuts, hazelnuts,

Nutrient	RDA	Food Sources
		oils (wheat germ, sunflower, walnut, safflower), asparagus
Phosphorus	1,000 mg	Beans (pinto, black, garbanzo, navy, lima, soy), rice and wheat bran, wheat germ, peas, tofu, corn
Vitamin B_{12}	2–3 mcg	B_{12} fortified soymilk and tofu, fortified cereals
Biotin	300 mcg	Soy flour, cereals, yeast

Oxygen Therapy

Every year, people with diabetes undergo approximately sixty thousand major amputations, most often of the toes, feet, and lower leg. These amputations are necessary because an infection has progressed to the point where gangrene has destroyed part of the limb. One way to prevent many of these devastating operations and to save limbs may be in the very air we breathe. Hyperbaric oxygen therapy *(hyper* means high; *baric* means atmosphere pressure), or HBO, is a controversial technique in which people inhale 100 percent oxygen in a pressurized environment. It is being used increasingly against several hard-to-treat conditions, such as foot ulcers and other poorly healing wounds in people with diabetes, burns, and bone infections.

Hyperbaric oxygen therapy isn't new. The technology was developed in the late 1800s to treat decompression sickness ("the bends") in deep-sea divers who returned to the surface too quickly. Recently its popularity as a therapy has been growing for conditions in which not enough oxygen gets to the tissues. Only 37 clinical decompression facilities were operating in the United States in 1977, and there are nearly 260 today. (There are two other forms of oxygen therapy: ozone therapy, which is highly controversial and not available in the United States; and hydrogen peroxide therapy, which has no application for diabetes. Information on these two approaches can be obtained by contacting the organizations listed in Appendix A.)

How Does Hyperbaric Oxygen Therapy Work?

The air we breathe contains 21 percent oxygen, which in most cases is sufficient for sustaining our life and allowing our bodies to heal themselves. If you have a wound that won't heal—for example, a diabetic foot ulcer—21 percent is not enough to promote healing. White blood cells need twenty times more oxygen when they are fighting and killing bacteria. If you have neuropathy (diabetic nerve damage; see Chapter 1), oxygen levels in your feet are probably low, which means healing is greatly slowed. A foot ulcer that doesn't heal may eventually require amputation of the toes or foot.

To get the amount of oxygen needed to heal wounds and avoid amputation, some individuals are stepping into a pressurized hyperbaric chamber and breathing 100-percent oxygen. The pressure in a hyperbaric chamber is the same as if you went scuba diving thirty-three feet under water. While in the chamber, you sit or lie down and breathe oxygen through a mask or head tent, or you may lie in a chamber that is pressured and filled with oxygen. In either case, it is the oxygen that you breathe in and is absorbed by your blood, and not that which touches your skin, that promotes healing.

After a treatment, oxygen levels remain high in the tissues for several hours. This promotes growth of new capillaries, which means more blood gets to the site of the wound and speeds up healing. Hyperbaric treatment also makes red blood cells more flexible so they flow more easily through the capillaries.

Oxygen Therapy for Diabetes

To stimulate healing of an ulcer or wound that is not infected, you will probably need treatment once a day for two hours for several weeks. These treatments can be done on an outpatient basis. If your wound is infected and there is a high risk of amputation, you will probably need two ninety-minute treatments a day for three to four weeks. Many cases of infected wounds require hospitalization and antibiotic treatment. If you take insulin, your physician may adjust your dose while you are in treatment.

According to Dr. John M. Alexander, director of the West Coast's largest civilian decompression facility at Northridge Hospital Medical Center, hyperbaric treatment, combined with a comprehensive wound-care program (tight blood glucose control, infection control with antibiotics, and good nutrition), could save up to half of the limbs now being amputated in people with diabetes and resolve about 70 percent of the wounds treated at his facility.

Is Hyperbaric Therapy for You?

If taken in excess, oxygen can cause toxic effects on the nervous system, resulting in grand mal (epileptic-type) seizures. This occurs in about one in ten thousand treatments and goes away once HBO treatment stops. Because HBO treatments are given in closed chambers, you may find it difficult or impossible to undergo treatment if you are claustrophobic. Fever and some medications can predispose you to oxygen seizures, so inform your doctor about what drugs you are taking.

To qualify for HBO therapy, you need good blood flow in the arteries of your feet. HBO therapy can be effective if you have deep ulcers that have extended into the bone or connective tissue, or if gangrene is present and you need amputation.

Polarity Therapy

Imagine your body is a battery, with the positive force at your head and the negative force at your feet. Now imagine five streams of energy flowing from your hands and feet and up through the top of your head through your body. These streams of energy are your vital force, and they flow along very specific pathways. This is what Dr. Randolph Stone, an osteopath, chiropractor, naturopath, and founder of polarity therapy believed, as do those who practice this therapy today. Polarity therapy is a healing technique based on the idea that health is linked with a smooth, vibrant flow of your vital force. Block that energy flow anywhere along the pathways and the result is imbalance. Dr. Stone described five energy centers in the body that he said must be in balance in order for the life force to flow unhindered (see Figure II-3, p. 186). To regain that balance, polarity therapists treat the energy flow, not the disease, and thus it is the energy that heals the body, not the therapist.

How Does Polarity Therapy Work?

Dr. Stone experimented with many different healing therapies before he put together what he believed are the best from the best: reflexology, craniosacral therapy (gentle manipulation of the bones in the head), deep massage, and Ayurvedic medicine (an Indian system of philosophy and medicine). Similar to other energy therapies, polarity therapy offers its healing powers by moving the vital force through sites where it is blocked. Polarity therapy may be especially beneficial for people with diabetes because of its holistic, three-part approach: body work (manipulation), stretching exercises, and nutrition, all of which address the three basic needs to be managed in good diabetes control. Thus nutrition, exercise, and stress management (body work) come together to restore healthy energy flow, relieve tension, and promote healing.

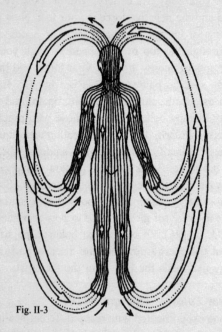

Fig. II-3

Polarity Therapy for Diabetes

The goal of polarity therapists is to help you learn self-treatment. This requires that you receive treatments from a professional therapist and/or learn the techniques and concepts from a workshop. During the body-work sessions, each of which typically lasts at least one hour, you will lie on a padded table, wearing loose clothing or just your underwear, either faceup or facedown to start. The practitioner will move his hands—one being positive and the other negative—over your body to different areas, pausing when he detects any blocked energy currents. When a blockage is found, he will move or release it, perhaps by grasping your hand or foot, applying deep pressure to the area, or rocking your arm, for example. Throughout the session, energy flows from one of the therapist's hands to the other and creates a current on your body, promoting the flow of your vital force.

Professional polarity therapists use three types of manipulations to release blocked energy:

- *Neutral:* light touches with the fingertips that soothe and balance the energy.
- *Positive:* application of light to medium pressure with the hands that is meant to move blocked energy.
- *Negative:* deep massage and pressure into the tissues, which can be painful.

Not all practitioners use deep massage, and those who do use it occasionally and selectively. Most people report feeling very relaxed or pleasantly tired after a polarity session.

The second aspect of polarity therapy is nutrition. Here, people with diabetes will need to pass on the polarity cleansing process, which involves fasting, and focus in on the primary diet recommended by polarity therapists, which is vegetarian. Included in this eating plan are all leafy and starchy vegetables, other vegetables and fruits, grains, sprouts, dairy (no eggs), and some sweets. Polarity therapists also stress the need to watch food combinations, as poor mixtures can cause poor absorption of nutrients by the body. Poor combinations include starches and proteins consumed together; dairy products, sweet fruits, and acidic fruits should be eaten alone. For more information, see the Suggested Reading List and Appendix A.

The third component of polarity therapy is stretching exercises. Your polarity therapist will teach you a series of movements that balance the currents of your vital flow, foster circulation, and help release toxins from your body.

Reflexology

Reflexology is an ancient holistic healing therapy in which pressure is applied to specific points on the hands and feet. These sites, called **reflex points,** are linked through your nervous system to other parts of your body. There are specific sites on your hands and feet, for example, that reflect the state of vital energy in your pancreas or pituitary gland, which have points you can work on for diabetes. When you or a reflexologist press or massage reflex points, the corresponding body part can respond by releasing blocked energy and toxins, increasing circulation, stimulating function of an organ, reducing stress, and promoting your body to heal itself.

You can do reflexology on yourself. We recommend, however, that you first have several sessions with a professional reflexologist so you can learn the different pressure-point techniques, where to press, and how much pressure to apply.

How Does Reflexology Work?

Theoretically, reflexology is similar to Oriental meridian therapies such as acupressure and acupuncture. All of these natural therapies are based on the holistic belief that any one part of the body reflects the whole. When you use reflexology to increase bioenergy flow, stimulate the circulation of blood and lymph in your body, and flush toxins out of your system, you are healing your entire body.

Reflexology can work two ways for you. One way is for you or a reflexologist to apply pressure to points that correspond specifically to your pancreas, adrenal glands, liver, pituitary, and thyroid. Application of pressure to these points (explained below) can stimulate the function of these organs and help reduce the risk of diabetic complications. If you are taking insulin—and even if you are not—and you are receiving reflexology treatment, monitor your blood glucose levels immediately after treatment and again twenty-four hours later. Treatments may stimulate your pancreas and reduce your insulin needs.

Another way you can benefit from reflexology is by having a complete foot or hand massage. This treatment can open up all of your body's reflex points and send a flood of healing energy throughout your body and promote relaxation and overall well-being. Many people say that a reflexology session that addresses all the points on their hands or feet is as relaxing as a complete body massage.

Reflexology Basics

Reflexology involves several different techniques to apply pressure or massage reflex points. Four you will need to know for the therapy we discuss are thumb-walking, finger-walking, pivoting, and sliding.

If you are using reflexology on yourself or someone is doing it to you, you are your own best judge of how much pressure is enough. Start with light pressure and increase it gradually. Practice on your own foot or that of a friend until you are comfortable with the techniques.

Thumb-walking is used on most of the reflex points in the hands and feet. To begin:

• Grasp the base of your big toe by placing your thumb on top and your index and middle fingers behind your toe.
• With the thumb bent at the first joint, allow only the outer edge of the thumb tip to be in contact with your toe as you "walk" your thumb toward the tip of your toe: press with your thumb, hold the press for several seconds, then release the pressure but do not lose contact with the toe.

Then move the thumb slightly forward and press again. Continue this routine until you reach the tip of your toe.

• Position your thumb so you avoid pressing your nail into the toe.

• Always keep your thumb joint bent.

Finger-walking is usually used on the top and sides of the feet and the back of the hands. You can use one, two, three, or four fingers for this technique, depending on which reflex you want to work. To begin the four-finger method:

• Place the tips of all four fingers on top of your foot close to your little toe. Keep all of the fingers bent, and keep your thumb on the side of your sole.

• Press with all four fingers, hold the press, and then release the pressure. Then move all four fingers together slightly down your foot toward your ankle and repeat the routine until you reach the base of your ankle.

Pivoting involves placing your thumb and fingers exactly as you do for thumb-walking. Instead of walking, however, you use your thumb to press on the reflex point you want to treat. Gently and slowly pivot your thumb on the point.

Reflexology for Diabetes

Now that you know a few basic techniques, you can prepare use them on some specific treatments. Find a comfortable, quiet place where you can sit undisturbed for about ten to fifteen minutes. Refer to Figures II-4 and II-5, pages 191 and 192, to help you with your sessions.

FOOT REFLEXOLOGY

To perform a complete foot reflexology session that touches on all of your reflex points:

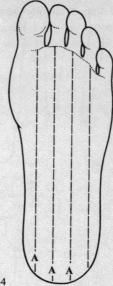

Fig. II-4

• Grasp the heel, toes, or ankle of your left foot with your left hand and place the thumb of your right hand on the sole of your foot at the heel. Using thumb-walking, start at point (A) and move toward your toes. When you reach the ball of your foot, return to the heel and start from a new spot (see the dotted lines).

• After you have covered your entire sole, massage the base pads and tips of all your toes and between the toes.

• Once you have completed work on the sole of your foot, use finger-walking on the top of the foot. Begin near your toes and work toward the base of your ankle. Use either two, three, or four fingers.

• Repeat the entire sequence on the other foot.

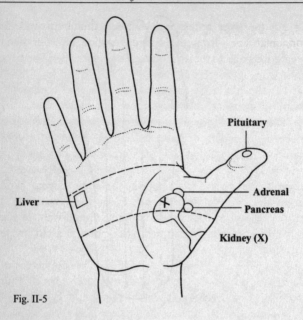

Fig. II-5

HAND REFLEXOLOGY

After you do the foot session above, you may want to try this hand session, which focuses on the specific organs to be strengthened in people with diabetes. The hand, as does the foot, has reflex points that correspond to the pancreas, adrenal glands, liver, pituitary gland, and kidney. Many people find it easier to do reflexology for specific points on their hands than on their feet, so we show you the reflex points for these organs in Figure II-5.

Work on each point for a few seconds and no more than a few minutes. As with any form of body work, leave a very tender point after you have done some gentle work and return to it after you have opened up other areas.

• For the **liver** reflex, use your left thumb to walk in horizontal lines from the outside portion of your hand toward the palm to the area marked in Figure II-5. The liver reflex is only on the right hand.

• For the **pancreas** reflex, thumb-walk from below the thumb of the right hand toward the palm.

• The **adrenal gland** reflex is found on both hands just above the waistline close to the kidney reflex. Use your thumb to rotate on this point in a clockwise direction.

• The **kidney** reflex is on both hands and is just above the adrenal-gland reflex. Beginning at the edge of your hand where the dotted line (referred to as the "waistline") crosses below the kidney reflex point, thumb-walk to the waistline and rotate around this reflex point in a clockwise direction.

• The **pituitary gland** reflex is located on the center of the fleshy part of your thumb. Use the outer edge of your thumb to gently rotate and press on the pituitary reflex.

Many people prefer reflexology over massage because it is more comfortable for them: it doesn't require them to get undressed or to have someone touching them except for their feet or hands. It is also safer for people who have conditions such as circulation problems for which it is best to avoid massage. Reflexology is an easy self-therapy and one that can be done while you're watching television or sitting in your office on break.

Tai Chi

Tai chi chuan (tai chi) is an ancient Chinese healing exercise that has been called the "Supreme Ultimate Exercise." It combines the Chinese philosophy of yang (positive) and yin (negative), the eternal opposites. When people do tai chi, they move from yin to yang (soft, slow, rest; to hard, fast, motion) and vice versa in harmonious balance. Tai chi is practiced in slow, graceful, dancelike motions, which makes it accessible to young and old, even those who have a physical disability or who are weak.

Traditional tai chi consists of more than a hundred different movements. It is not necessary to learn them all, and you do not need to follow the motions exactly in order to reap the benefits. It is best, however, to learn the basic moves from a professional tai chi practitioner (see Appendix A). When you do, you also will learn how tai chi is both a physical and mental healing exercise. To help illustrate this connection, instructors often suggest that students use colorful imagery. They may suggest that you "move like a swan" or "push with your hands as if you were moving the wind." Such visual images are part of tai chi and can help increase your awareness of the mind/body connection.

Before beginning tai chi, consult with your doctor. You may also want to inform your tai chi instructor that you have diabetes if you have any concerns about hypoglycemia or any other medical condition. Whether you go to a class or do tai chi at home, dress for the occasion: wear light, loose clothing—sweat clothes are good—and tennis or aerobic shoes. Avoid heels or shoes with hard soles.

How Tai Chi Works

Tai chi consists of gentle, steady movements that follow the way the body is designed to move. It has attracted much attention in the medical community because of the benefits it has demonstrated. Tai chi requires that you relax the muscles of the wrist, arms, shoulders, chest, back, and abdomen. This relaxation contributes to feelings of peace and calm. The muscular relaxation causes the blood vessels to expand, which in turn lowers blood pressure and helps prevent arteriosclerosis. Tai chi breathing is deep and rhythmic, which stimulates blood circulation in the stomach and intestines.

Regular practice of tai chi helps maintain overall good health and prevents kidney deficiency, or what the Chinese call *shun shi*. According to traditional Chinese medicine, shun shi is a sign of overall weakness in the body. Elderly people who practice tai chi do not have *shun shi,* while about half of those who were inactive did. Tai chi also helps improve the functioning of the nervous and digestive systems and helps keep bones and joints in good condition.

Tai Chi for Diabetes

Tai chi movements are usually performed in an order that allows one movement to flow naturally into the next. To experience an entire sequence of movements, you will need to take a class or refer to one of the books listed in the Bibliography and Suggested Reading. Here, we give you an idea of what tai chi is all about by explaining two warm-up movements and the first two of a series of tai chi movements.

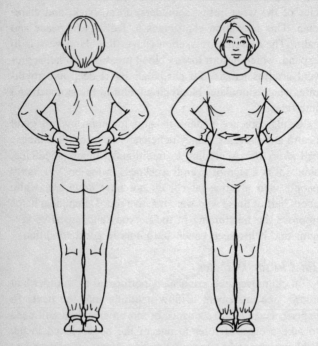

Fig. II-6

WARM-UP 1

• Stand straight with your feet together and your knees straight but not locked. Place your hands on your waist with your fingers pointed toward the small of your back and your thumbs forward.

• Push your stomach forward with your fingers.

• Use a circular motion and rotate your waist thirty-two times to the right and thirty-two times to the left.

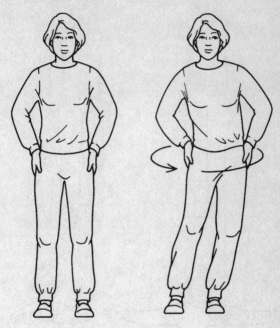

Fig. II-7

WARM-UP 2

• Stand straight with your feet parallel and about one foot apart.

• Place your hands on your sides of your lower hip. Your thumbs should face forward while your fingers point back and down.

• With your left hand, push your hip toward the right and rotate your hips in an oval pattern thirty-two times to the right and thirty-two times to the left.

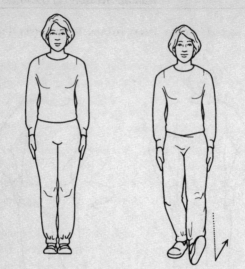

Fig. II-8

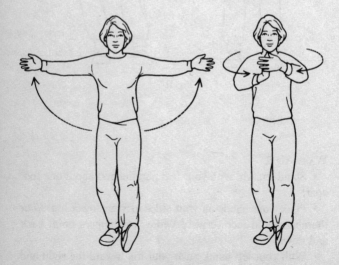

Fig. II-9

MOVEMENT 1: STRIKE PALM TO ASK BUDDHA (SEE FIGURE II-8)

- Stand straight, feet together and hands to your sides.
- Turn your right foot to the right forty-five degrees.
- Bend both knees slightly and move your left foot forward about two feet. Keep your left knee straight, your heel on the ground, and your toes pointed up.
- Raise both arms in front of you to shoulder level and face palms forward.
- While keeping your arms up, bring your hands together until they almost touch. Your hands should be about eighteen inches from your chest.
- Keeping your hands open, bend the right hand at the wrist so that it is perpendicular to the middle of the left hand. Hold this position for several seconds before you move on to the next movement.

MOVEMENT 2: GRASP BIRD'S TAIL (SEE FIGURE II-9)

- From the ending position of movement 1 (with your arms still up), move your left foot back past your right heel to the left until it is forty-five degrees in back of your right foot. Your left foot should be perpendicular to your right foot and the right toes should point up.
- Move your hands down to waist level and diagonal to your left hip. Keep both elbows bent slightly, your left palm up and the right palm down. Your right leg should be straight and the toes up.
- Bring your right leg back until the ball of the right foot touches the arch of the left foot.
- Step forward and diagonally with your right foot. Bend both knees and center your weight. Keep your back straight.
- Twist at the waist and shoulder until your hands are even.

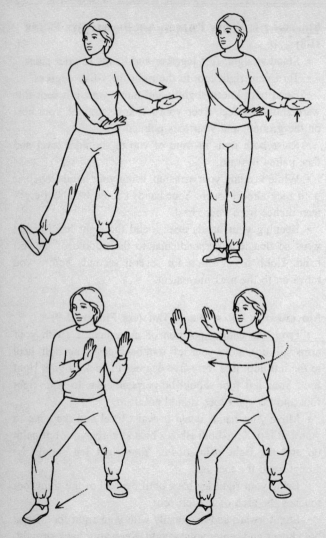

Fig. II-10

Tips for Doing Tai Chi (see Figure II-10)

• Practice every day.

• Every movement must include the entire body. It takes time to remember to move your right and left hands at the same time or to move your legs and arms simultaneously.

• Breathe naturally, deeply, and with your abdomen. Do not pant or hold your breath. When first learning tai chi, it is common to have trouble coordinating your movements with your breathing. As you become proficient in different movements, you will synchronize the two.

• Keep your body relaxed and your posture natural. Do not hold the military stance: chest out, buttocks out. Instead, relax the waist, abdomen, and chest muscles.

• Tai chi is an internal movement as well as an external, physical one. Visualize each movement as you do it. It may help to keep your eyes closed partly or completely. When you visualize your movements in your mind, you create agreement between what you are doing and what you are thinking, and this in turn promotes inner harmony.

• Concentrate on your movements; avoid distractions.

• Keep your knees bent slightly whenever your body is in motion.

• Keep your movements fluid and without tension.

Visualization and Guided Imagery

Visualization and guided imagery are two similar types of meditation in which you focus on or create images of people, places, situations, or things in your mind to help you achieve a specific goal. The goal may be to stimulate blood circulation, relieve muscle tension, improve your immune system, or lower your blood pressure, for example. During **visualization,** you enter a very relaxed state and totally focus your attention on one or more images you hold in your mind's eye. This can be a scene you find particularly relaxing, such as a deserted beach, a meadow full of flowers, or a church. Some individuals imagine themselves seated with God or Buddha; others picture themselves surrounded by a white, healing light. What's important is that the image you choose is meaningful and calming for you. This image is your own special place.

Guided imagery is a technique you can use to take a mental "trip" through your scene. This technique is similar to creating an entire story in your mind and in which you can use all of your senses, if you choose to do so, rather than just vision. Therefore, instead of just picturing yourself in a meadow, you can also smell the flowers, hear the birds fly overhead, and feel the grass brush against your legs.

Guided imagery and hypnotherapy are sometimes used together, although they are two independent techniques (see "Hypnosis"). In hypnosis, you induce a particular static state of mind, while in **imagery** (the term we use throughout this section for both visualization or guided imagery), you actively participate in the state you create.

You can learn imagery on your own from self-help books or tapes, or you can study with someone who gives private or group sessions. Sources of help with imagery can be found in appendices A and B.

How Does Imagery Work?

A growing number of physicians are using imagery to help their patients deal with stress or chronic disease such as diabetes and cancer, and they are seeing significant results. Integrative guided imagery has even been chosen to be part of the required curriculum for medical students in the Integrative Medicine Program at the University of Arizona College of Medicine, directed by Dr. Andrew Weil.

It is difficult, however, to conduct well-controlled studies of how imagery works. One problem is that each person's imaging powers and techniques are unique, so standard measuring methods are impossible to develop. Another reason is that imagery is usually used along with other mind/body therapies, such as hypotherapy or meditation, which makes it hard to determine the impact of each technique alone.

Using a brain scanning technique called positron emission tomography (PET), researchers have discovered that certain parts of the brain are activated whether you imagine you are experiencing something or you actually do experience it. For example, whether you imagine you are eating a juicy lemon or actually bite into one, the same area of your brain will be activated. This finding leads many researchers to believe that the more vividly you imagine something, especially by using as many senses as possible, the more you will activate your brain cells and your nervous system.

Imagery for Diabetes

According to Martin L. Rossman, M.D., author of *Healing Yourself: A Step-by-Step Program for Better Health Through Imagery,* there are many imagery approaches you can use to promote healing at some level, regardless of the ailment. One approach is called "Turning Insight into Action," which is a way to make dietary, physical, attitudinal, and lifestyle changes that can improve your health. Because committing to a movement therapy program is often difficult, you may want to use that goal in the following imagery exercise on how to turn insight into action. Feel free to use whatever insight or goal you choose.

To do this imagery exercise, you will need to have paper and a writing utensil at hand. If you wish, tape the session so you can use it again and again.

Get into a comfortable sitting position with your writing materials near at hand. . . . Your eyes will remain open during much of this session until you reach mental rehearsal. . . .

You will now begin the process of grounding. The process has been broken down into steps for you. . . . This will allow you to make changes happen based on the insights you reach. . . .

First, you need to *clarify* your insight or goal. . . . Take some time to state for yourself what you want to act on. . . . [routine movement program] Write the statement down in the clearest terms possible. . . . [I want to begin and maintain a regular exercise routine four days a week for at least thirty minutes each session] . . . Carefully read the statement to yourself and decide which word or phrase is the most important one. . . . [regular exercise routine] . . . Decide if this word or phrase is the one that best describes what you want to accomplish; if not, choose another word. . . .

Second, *think about your goal* and how you might make it happen—do some brainstorming to help you. . . . Write down as many possibilities you can think of, even if they aren't realistic or practical. . . . [take up jogging, join an aerobics class after work, buy a stationary bike, purchase a membership in the health club, walk with my friend Judy in the morning before work]

Read over your options. . . . Which ones are practical? Which ones would be easy to do? Is there one that you feel very comfortable with or that excites you?

Next, *choose* the option that makes the most sense for you . . . highlight or circle that choice . . . [walk with Judy]

Now, *affirm* your choice. . . . Do whatever you need to do to make your choice real for you. . . . Say it aloud: "I choose to walk with Judy on Mondays, Tuesdays, Thursdays, and Saturdays.'' . . . Write this statement down several times to make it real for you. . . .

The next step is to *make a firm plan* to follow through on your choice: . . . Think about what steps you need to take to get started: . . . Keep it simple yet specific so you will follow through. . . . [call Judy and plan to meet her on Saturday, buy walking shoes, learn some easy stretching exercises for warm-up]

Next, *rehearse your plan in your mind.* . . . Close your eyes and take a few slow, deep breaths. . . . With each exhalation release any thoughts in your mind. . . . With each inhalation take in energy . . . with each exhalation send your tensions to the universe. . . . now breathe gently and easily. . . . Allow your mind to be quiet. . . . You may want to imagine yourself in your own special place. . . . once you feel completely relaxed, imagine yourself carrying out your plan. . . . picture yourself carrying out the activity from start to finish. . . . [putting on your shoes, doing your stretching exercises, meeting Judy on the corner, walking along the path, swinging your arms and breathing deeply, talking with Judy, parting company after the walk] . . . As you go on your imaginary journey, notice if there are any obstacles to your plan. . . . [a rainy day, Judy is sick] . . . Imagine how you will adjust your plan to accommodate these obstacles. . . . [plan to walk in an enclosed mall instead, find another friend to join you] . . . Imagine yourself carrying out your plan with the changes. . . . Repeat your rehearsal, imagining that your plan goes off without a hitch. . . . Keep rehearsing your plan until you feel comfortable with it. . . . Bring in all your senses to make it more real for you. . . . [smell the flowers, feel the breeze, hear the birds, create a conversation between yourself and Judy] . . .

When you are ready, open your eyes slowly and take

some time to come back to consciousness. . . . Write
down any obstacles you came across during your imaginary journey and note how you will take care of them.
. . . Feel empowered to act on your plans!

All that's left at this point is to carry out your plans. You
may encounter problems or obstacles you did not anticipate
during your imagery session. If so, you may want to do
another imagery session and focus on that obstacle alone,
or you may decide to choose a whole new activity. In any
case, you now have a tool to help you make positive,
healthy changes to your lifestyle.

Although many people with diabetes use imagery to help
them eliminate or reduce stress and thus maintain better
control of their glucose levels, some people can do even
more than that. According to Belleruth Naparstek *(Staying
Well with Guided Imagery),* you can use imagery to get
glucose from your blood into your cells. This type of imagery is called ''cellular imagery,'' and can be used to
work directly on insulin and glucose in the body. Specially
designed cellular imagery audiotapes for diabetes as well as
its complications, such as hypertension and heart disease,
are available in the *Health Journeys* series, through Image
Paths, Inc. (see Appendix B).

The imagery session below is a much abbreviated adapta-
tion of one from *Staying Well with Guided Imagery* and is
similar to a cellular imagery session. It may help reduce
blood pressure, maintain healthy blood vessels, and metabolize blood glucose. We suggest you tape this session so
you can use it again and again. Pause at the appropriate
spots. Please feel free to embellish upon this version to suit
your own needs.

Lie down on a comfortable surface so your body is
aligned and you feel relaxed. Remove restrictive clothing.

Take a deep, full, cleansing breath. . . . Inhale as completely as you can . . . (pause) . . . and exhale completely. . . . (pause) . . .

Take in another complete breath. . . . Breathe into your belly if you can . . . (pause) . . . and exhale completely. . . . (pause) . . .

Again, breathe in deeply. . . . send your breath into any part of your body where you feel tense or sore. . . . As you exhale release that feeling. . . . Notice that with each inhalation you feel looser, softer, and more relaxed. . . .

If any stray thoughts enter your mind . . . send them away as you exhale. . . . Release them so your mind is free. . . .

Focus on your body. . . . Feel your blood moving through your veins. . . . You may feel it pulse. . . . You may hear it vibrate . . . sense its warmth. . . . In your mind's eye you may see the miniature highways that crisscross throughout your body. . . . Acknowledge this intricate system of life. . . . (pause) . . .

Feel the blood expand your veins and arteries, making them flexible and strong . . . keeping them clean and smooth . . . never allowing debris to hinder the flow. . . .

Feel as the blood strengthens any weak spots in the arteries. . . . Feel as the blood repairs them and fills them with nourishment. . . . Sense how the blood flow reduces any debris that may have gathered. . . . Experience the rush of rich blood as it gently carries the debris away. . . . Feel how smooth and clean the blood vessels are. . . . Sense the blood flowing through your body down to your toes. . . .

Allow the blood to reach freely into the smallest places. . . . Know that it is dissolving any debris. . . . turning it into tiny specks until they disappear. . . .

Feel as your blood feeds your tissues. . . . Sense how the glucose and nutrients in the blood are soaked up by your hungry cells. . . . Feel your cells eagerly fill up with glucose. . . . Sense your body regaining power and energy. . . .

Feel the incredible power of this new awareness . . . thankful for the healing . . . grateful for the strength and resilience you feel. . . .

Slowly return to your surroundings. . . . Take a deep, full breath. . . . Gradually open your eyes. . . . Return to the place from where you began . . . knowing you are better for this. . . . And so you are. . . .

Yoga

Yoga is an ancient Eastern Indian philosophy and science of inner harmony, health, and well-being that is rapidly gaining acceptance and popularity in Western cultures. There are many types of yoga, yet they share several common elements: they slow down breathing, relax the muscles, and calm the mind. When you combine and practice these three techniques in a yogic tradition, you can achieve inner harmony, reduce stress, and enjoy many other health benefits, which we discuss here.

Yoga therapy can be used to treat many conditions, including diabetes, and its complications, such as heart disease, hypertension, obesity, depression, and poor circulation. In this section we will show you how you can stretch, strengthen, and heal your body using gentle movements and postures while you focus your mind on your breathing and physical sensations. These approaches allow your body and mind to work together to heal, which makes yoga a true mind/body approach to health.

How Does Yoga Work?

More than two thousand years ago, Patanjali, who wrote the classic book on yoga, called this ancient method "a science of the mind." Yoga is a way of life: a technique to achieve physical, emotional, and spiritual health. It offers you a way to control your mind and your reactions to stressful situations. It allows you to fully focus your attention on an object or a subject and to quiet the "noise" in your mind. With practice, you can achieve inner peace at all times in your life. This is sometimes referred to as "calmness in action" and helps you maintain physical and mental health.

To be effective, you need to practice yoga daily. People with diabetes who have made yoga a part of their lives find that it moderates their blood glucose and blood pressure levels and rewards them with a sense of well-being and calm. Some people claim it also has helped them lose weight.

Yoga for Diabetes

Yoga is a powerful complementary therapy for people receiving conventional medical treatment for diabetes. Practiced regularly, yoga can help regulate blood glucose levels, reduce stress-hormone levels, tone the body, help with weight control, improve the function of the pancreas, and strengthen the immune system. In individuals with Type II diabetes, it can eliminate or reduce the need for insulin or oral hypoglycemic drugs. People with Type I diabetes may experience a reduced insulin requirement or better control of insulin levels, although yoga cannot eliminate the need for insulin.

Before you start yoga, consult with your physician. We recommend that you seek out a good yoga instructor (see Appendix A for assistance). Although you can learn postures from a book, it is most helpful to take a few lessons so you can experience firsthand proper breathing, meditation, and simple postures. Also, it is best to work with a yoga instructor who has experience teaching individuals with diabetes.

All yoga sessions, regardless of whether you have diabetes or not, begin with a basic warm-up format. The warm-up portion consists of breath exercises, stretching, and loosening-up postures. These exercises calm you and prepare you for the *asanas,* postures that help you relax and tone your muscles and massage your internal organs. Asanas also improve breathing and circulation, and on a subtle level also release your vital energy flow. The asanas and any special postures you do for diabetes or other ailments are followed by a time for relaxation. After relaxation you practice *pranayama,* which are breathing exercises that slow your breathing and regulate the flow of energy, or *prana,* through your body. You end your yoga session with meditation, which calms your mind and spirit. In this section we discuss a few of the postures. Breathing, relaxation, and meditation are discussed at length elsewhere in this book. Good nutrition is also an important part of yoga and is discussed in its own section as well.

It is not within the scope of this book to present all the possible yoga postures for diabetes; that would prove to be too extensive. See the Bibliography and Suggested Reading for some excellent books that discuss yoga and diabetes. We can, however, offer you a sample of what to expect and a few yoga postures that are generally recommended for people with diabetes. Your own program will differ, however, depending on your physical condition and any medical ailments you may have, so work with your instructor and physician. Also, read "Preparing for Yoga" on pages 211–212.

PREPARING FOR YOGA

• Before you begin a yoga program, consult your physician so you both can assess your flexibility and any conditions that may limit your ability to do some yoga postures. If you are pregnant or have a back problem, for example, there are some postures you should avoid.

• Wear comfortable clothes that allow you to see what your body is doing. Shorts and a T-shirt, leotards, or a swimsuit are fine; sweatpants are not.

• Bare feet are the rule.

• Have the following props with you:

• Head and neck support rolls (folded or rolled-up hand towels for the neck; bath towel for the head).

• Lumbar pad (folded bath towel).

• Blankets (wool or heavy cotton are best).

• A nonskid mat if you are doing your postures on a nonskid floor. It's important to properly align your head, neck, and back, so experiment with the placement and thickness of the rolls and pads until you are comfortable.

• To reap the most benefit from your yoga sessions, you need to breathe properly.

• Inhale and exhale through your nose.

• As you inhale, relax the muscles in your face, neck, and shoulders and focus on maintaining correct posture.

• As you exhale, perform the action of the pose.

• Never hold your breath.

• If you focus on your breathing during your yoga sessions, you bring in the benefits of meditation—stress reduction and increased self-awareness.

• Make meditation a part of your daily routine. Set aside fifteen to thirty minutes a day, at least five days a week, for yoga. If fifteen to thirty minutes it not always possible, spend whatever time you can; something is better than nothing.

Yoga for Diabetes: Warm-up—Breathe and Stretch

Of the half dozen or so breathing and stretching warm-up exercises, the **arm-stretch breathing** and **hand-stretch breathing** are the easiest and generally safe for everyone. When you do these and any other breathe-and-stretch exercises:

- Keep your eyes closed.
- Focus on your inner sensations as you breathe.
- Exhale for a longer count than you inhale: for example, if you inhale to a count of six, exhale to a count of eight or ten.

ARM-STRETCH BREATHING

Stand straight with your feet together. Stretch your arms out in front of you at shoulder height and put your palms together. As you inhale, spread your arms out to your sides and expand your chest. When you are ready to exhale, bring your arms back to the front, still at shoulder height. Synchronize your breathing and arm movements so you finish the inhalation when your arms are fully outstretched to your sides and you finish the exhalation when your arms are back front.

HAND-STRETCH BREATHING

Stand straight with your feet together. Place your hands on your chest with your fingers interlinked and palms facing inward. As you inhale, stretch out your arms to the front at shoulder level and flip your hands so the palms face outward. As you exhale, bring your hands back to your chest to the starting position. Repeat three times. Then do the same movement again, only this time extend your arms at a forty-five-degree angle upward. After doing this three times, repeat the movement again; this time bring your arms up above your head. Repeat three times.

AN ASANA FOR DIABETES

When you do asanas, be aware of how your body feels: experience each stretch and any changes in pressure. Allow yourself to relax into the posture as you exhale and hold the position as you inhale. Never strain or exert yourself to reach or maintain a position; relaxation is the key.

The **spinal twist** is recommended for people with diabetes, but avoid it if you have disk problems. To do the spinal twist:

• Sit on the floor with your legs stretched out in front of you. Raise your right leg and place your right foot to the left of your left knee.

• Exhale and turn your torso to the right.

• Bring your left arm over and to the right of your upright knee and grasp your right shin, if you can.

• Gradually move your hand down your leg until you can grasp your ankle. If you can't reach your ankle, go as far as you can comfortably.

• Rest your right hand on the floor behind you and keep your back straight.

• Remember to keep your exhalations longer than your inhalations.

• Each time you exhale, twist a bit farther to the right. Use your arms to help you, but don't strain.

• After three or four exhalations, slowly return to the starting position and do the same posture for the other side: that is, raise your left leg and place your left foot to the right of your right knee, and so on.

SPECIAL POSTURE FOR DIABETES

Yoga has many special postures that aid in the healing of various conditions. For diabetes, a posture called **abdominal pumping** massages the internal organs. To do this posture:

• Stand with your knees slightly bent and your hands resting on your knees.

• Lean forward and exhale completely through your mouth. Close your throat so no air can get into your lungs.

• Expand your chest as if you were inhaling and suck your abdomen up into your chest.

• With your lungs still empty, relax your stomach muscles so your abdomen comes out.

• To do the pumping motion, suck in your abdomen again and then release it. Keep repeating this in-and-out motion until you need to inhale.

• Breathe normally. Then repeat the pumping motion for three more rounds, resting when you need to inhale again.

• Warning: Avoid this posture if you are pregnant, menstruating, or have heart disease or hypertension.

RELAXATION

There are several relaxation techniques in yoga; we present one of them here. Relaxation postures can be done after individual exercises or anytime during the day when you feel stressed or need a rest. Whenever you do a relaxation posture, always come out of it slowly.

To begin relaxation, get into the **corpse pose.** To do so:

• Lie flat and faceup on a firm surface. To reduce the space between your lower back and the floor, lift your knees to your chest and then slide your feet along the floor as you lower your legs.

• Let your feet rest about ten to twelve inches apart on the floor.
• Spread your arms out to your sides so they are about eighteen inches from your body. Keep your palms up.
• If your neck is uncomfortable, put a cushion under your head or rest your head on its side.
• Close your eyes.

You are now ready to do a relaxation exercise.

• Focus on how your body feels on the floor. Notice how your abdomen and chest rise and fall as you breathe.
• Count ten cycles of breathing. Notice the rhythm of your breath.
• Count another ten cycles of breathing and feel your breath going into your abdomen. Do not force your breathing.
• For the next cycle, focus on each exhalation. Feel yourself relax more and more with each exhalation.
• Experience a feeling of lightness as you inhale.
• Feel your body sink into the floor as your abdomen falls.
• Repeat this cycle ten times.

Remember to get up slowly after each relaxation session.
Yoga can provide you with physical, emotional, and spiritual balance and well-being. Once you learn a few basic stretches and postures, you can add to your sessions as you go. Always consult with a member of your health-care team to be sure any new postures you add will complement your diabetes management program.

PART THREE

MEDICAL THERAPY FOR DIABETES

Diabetes is a chronic, life-threatening disease that, in many cases, requires some level of medical intervention at some point during the course of the disease. This is certainly true for people with Type I diabetes, who need insulin to stay alive. Along with the use of insulin in Type I diabetes, and insulin or diabetes pills, or both, in some individuals with Type II diabetes, many people with diabetes develop complications that require treatment.

In this section, we discuss two categories of medical intervention for people with diabetes. First are items related directly to blood glucose control, including the different types of insulin, insulin pumps, and diabetes pills; how they are used, their benefits, and side effects. Second, we discuss some of the medical interventions available to those with diabetic complications, such as retinopathy, neuropathy, kidney disease, and blood vessel disease.

The information in this section is not intended to be used as medical advice. Consult your physician and management team before you make any change to your current management program.

Insulin

Before insulin was first extracted from the pancreas of animals in 1921 and injected into animals with diabetes, most people with Type I diabetes died, and those with Type II lived limited lives. But within a year of these experiments with insulin, conducted by physicians Charles Best and Frederick Banting, animal insulin was being administered to humans.

Today, insulin is produced in two ways. The lesser-used type is still extracted from the pancreas of pigs or cows, but this type can cause allergic reactions in some people. The more popular version is produced in laboratories by bacteria that are "programmed," through genetic engineering, to make synthetic human insulin. All insulin must be taken by injection, or through a pump, rather than by mouth, because it is a protein and would be destroyed by stomach acids if ingested.

Types of Insulin

There are nearly thirty types of insulin, which fall into three broad categories: short- (Regular), intermediate- (NPH and Lente), and long-acting (Ultralente) (see Table III-1). Insulin works by helping glucose enter the walls of your cells so it can be used as energy. **Exogenous** insulins (meaning those that are introduced into the body, as opposed to **endogenous** insulin, which is produced naturally by the body) all differ in how quickly they start to work, when they reach their peak activity in the body, and how long they will continue to work. This wide selection allows people with diabetes the advantage of mixing and matching types according to their unique needs. Some types of insulin can be purchased premixed—one short- and one intermediate-acting together, for example. The benefit of such a mixture is that it gives your body one insulin that will act immediately as well as one that will start acting when the first one is through. This eliminates the need for a second injection.

TABLE III-1
ACTIVITY OF INSULIN TYPES

	Short-Acting	Intermediate-Acting	Long-Acting
Starts Working Within	30 min	1–3 hrs	4–5 hrs
Activity Peak	2–4 hrs	6–12 hrs	12–18 hrs
Duration of Activity	6–8 hrs	18–26 hrs	24–48 hrs

Choosing Your Insulin

You and your management team will work together to determine your insulin requirements. Establishing the exact schedule for your particular needs often takes trial and error. If you have Type I diabetes, the stage of disease you are in (see Chapter 1) has a great impact on the type and timing of your insulin doses. Other factors include your weight and level of physical activity.

Some people with Type II diabetes take insulin injections because meal planning, exercise, and diabetes pills have not been successful in stabilizing their blood glucose levels. Sometimes beta cells become defective or are partially destroyed in Type II disease. If any of these situations occur, your physician may prescribe insulin. The exact amount and timing of injections vary greatly from person to person. Some people take both insulin and diabetes pills. Your specific needs can change over time, depending on how well you follow your meal plan, movement therapy program, stress management, and medication schedule.

Choosing an Insulin Therapy Approach

For the approximately eight hundred thousand people with Type I diabetes, daily doses of insulin are their lifeline. Among the 8 million people diagnosed with Type II diabetes, about 30 percent use insulin for blood glucose control. If you need to take insulin, the type, dose, and timing of injections are all decided by you and your doctor, based on periodic readings taken of your blood glucose levels during a twenty-four-hour period.

For many years, people who need insulin therapy have had to anticipate their insulin needs over the next six to twelve hours and inject the appropriate amount of insulin based on their projected activity level and food intake. The result is an insulin schedule that consists of one to three injections of "fixed" doses that are given at a set time each day. This requires these individuals to maintain a somewhat predictable lifestyle and be prepared for any significant change that may lead to a hypoglycemic episode.

Since the DCCT results were announced, more physicians are opting for a tight control approach for blood glucose. This method requires a bit more work on your part: If you have Type I diabetes, tight control means you'll take three or four shots daily or use an insulin pump (see pp. 224–225) and monitor your blood glucose levels more often. However, it allows you and others with flexible lifestyles to vary your insulin doses according to your activities on any given day. For people with Type II disease, experts are recommending more careful and frequent monitoring.

Using Insulin

Insulin is injected into the fatty tissue beneath the skin, usually of the abdomen, upper buttocks, front of the legs, or back of the arms, using a syringe. Insulin is measured in "units," and is designated by the letter *U*. Most people in the United States use a "100" strength insulin—U-100—

which means the dose contains a hundred units of insulin in each cubic centimeter of liquid. You must use a U-100 syringe to administer this strength of insulin. In other countries, different strengths may be available, so be aware if you are traveling.

Insulin enters the bloodstream fastest through the abdomen and more slowly in the thighs and hips. Your nurse educator or physician will teach you how to measure and inject the correct dose of insulin for your needs and to determine how to rotate injection sites.

The secret to good blood glucose control is timing your insulin injections so the insulin begins to work when the glucose from the food you eat starts to enter your bloodstream. Careful monitoring of your blood glucose levels throughout the day and comparing them with your activities will give you and your management team the information needed to develop the best medication schedule for you.

Injection Devices

Several types of syringes are available to inject insulin. Some require you to insert the needle into your skin and push the plunger. Others have automatic injectors, which are equipped with a spring. When you place the injector against your skin, you push a trigger and the needle enters your skin. You then push the plunger down to inject the insulin. If you can't tolerate needles, you may use a jet injector, which uses great pressure to drive insulin through your skin. Another alternative is to use an insulin pump. In the development stage is a patch that will deliver insulin through the skin, similar to how a nicotine patch works, except the insulin patch is equipped with a tiny ultrasound pump.

Precautions

Here are some general precautions to consider when taking insulin.

• Other drugs can have an effect on insulin by either increasing or decreasing its effect. Drugs that can decrease insulin's efficacy include anticonvulsants, oral contraceptives, cortisone, diuretics, furosemide, and thyroid medications.

• Drugs that can increase insulin's impact include oral antidiabetics, MAO inhibitors, antismoking preparations that contain nicotine, oxyphenbutazone, phenylbutazone, bismuth subsalicylate, sulfa drugs, tetracyclines, and any drugs that contain aspirin.

• Use of beta-blockers may make blood glucose control difficult and also may hide any warning signs of hypoglycemic shock.

• Generally, alcohol is best avoided, as it can cause hypoglycemia.

• Regular smoking can decrease your body's ability to absorb insulin and increase your need for insulin by about 30 percent.

• Do not stop taking insulin or change the type you are taking without first consulting your physician.

Insulin Pumps

An insulin infusion pump is a device about the size of a beeper that slowly but continuously releases insulin to the body tissues through tubing and a needle. The needle is inserted under the fat, usually in the abdomen, and taped into place. The device can be worn on your belt or inside a pocket.

Current infusion pumps use only regular insulin. They can be set to deliver a constant flow of insulin as well as a burst of insulin over a few seconds before meals. Use of an insulin pump is not necessarily easier than injecting insulin, because it does require you to monitor your blood glucose levels more often. The pump also allows you to easily make adjustments to your insulin needs as they change.

Use of an insulin pump is not for everyone. For some people, delivery of a constant supply of regular insulin gives them better glucose control than does injections of intermediate- or long-acting insulin. Some people appear to have difficulty absorbing and utilizing these two insulin types, which leads to poor blood glucose control. An insulin pump often can provide them with the control they need.

An alternative to an external insulin pump is an implantable pump, which should be available commercially in the near future. These pumps are implanted in a pocket surgically created in the abdominal wall and have a reservoir that must be refilled every one to three months, depending on your insulin needs. A handheld programmer is used to communicate with the pump and adjust insulin delivery. Since 1980, more than 780 pumps have been implanted in people with diabetes. Improvement in blood glucose control has not been accompanied by an increase in incidences of severe hypoglycemia, and user satisfaction has been good. At least initially, cost of implantable pumps will be high (estimated range, $10,000 to $15,000 plus surgical costs), and, based on current technology, they will need to be replaced after several years.

Diabetes Pills

Most people with Type II diabetes use diabetes pills (also referred to as oral agents) at some time during the course of their disease. Diabetes pills are taken in addition to, and not in place of, exercise and a sound eating plan. Some doctors recommend diabetes pills if, despite their patients' efforts to lose weight, exercise regularly, and stay with a healthy eating plan, they cannot obtain and maintain good blood-glucose control. Diabetes pills are also usually recommended over insulin in obese people with Type II diabetes, because overweight individuals generally need large doses of insulin, and insulin can stimulate weight gain even more than some diabetes pills do. Diabetes pills are also easier to take than insulin, and they cause fewer hypoglycemic reactions.

Other physicians, like John McDougall, M.D., medical director of St. Helena Hospital in Deer Park, California (see "McDougall Program" under "Nutrition" in Part II), believe diabetes pills should be avoided because of their side effects. Regular use of diabetes pills, for example, increases the risk of dying from heart disease by 2.5 times more than among diabetics who control their disease by diet alone. They also contribute to obesity by causing excess calories to be stored in the fat cells.

How Do Diabetes Pills Work?

Diabetes pills are prescribed primarily to stimulate the pancreas to release insulin. They also are designed to act on your cells in several ways. One way is to reduce your cells' resistance to insulin and allow your body to more efficiently use the insulin your body produces. Another way is to increase the sensitivity of the insulin receptors on your cells, which allows your body to function efficiently on low amounts of insulin. Diabetes pills also prevent the liver from releasing too much glucose into the bloodstream, which can result in hyperglycemia.

Types of Diabetes Pills

There are three classes of oral agents to control diabetes: sulfonylureas, biguanides, and alpha-glucosidase inhibitors. All but one drug are for use in people with Type II diabetes only. The one exception, the alpha-glucosidase, acarbose, may be taken in addition to, but *not* in place of, insulin in people with Type I diabetes. We discuss the three classes of diabetes pills here.

SULFONYLUREAS (SUL-FA-NIL-YUR-EE-AHS)

The most commonly used diabetes pills are sulfonylureas, which have been available in the United States for more than forty years. Sulfonylureas stimulate the pancreas to produce more insulin, thus lowering the blood glucose level. They also may enhance the sensitivity of the body's tissues and make them more receptive to insulin.

Sulfonylureas are available in three strengths: short-, intermediate-, and long-acting. This means the drug remains working in your body for either up to twelve, thirty, or sixty hours before you need another dose. You and your physician will determine which type of sulfonylurea will best suit your needs.

Use of sulfonylureas can cause many side effects. Most sulfonylureas are broken down by the liver and excreted by the kidneys. If you have liver or kidney problems, you need to avoid the sulfonylureas that are processed in this way (see list pp. 228–229). Sulfonylureas may cause you to gain weight, but usually not as much as you might if you used insulin. If you are allergic to sulfa drugs, your doctor may prescribe another diabetes pill, as sulfonylureas may cause an allergic reaction. Also avoid using these drugs if you are pregnant, have an infection or injury, have recently undergone surgery, or are taking long-term corticosteroid therapy. Use of sulfonylureas may cause hypoglycemia, fatigue, indigestion, nausea and vomiting, and liver damage.

After about three months of continual treatment with sufficient doses, sulfonylureas lose their effectiveness in 40 percent of people. Among individuals who initially get good control with sulfonylureas, between 25 and 30 percent will lose that control over time. Routine follow-up examinations are necessary to evaluate treatment programs that include sulfonylureas. Once one sulfonylurea is no longer effective, your physician may prescribe another or switch you to metformin (see p. 229).

Below are descriptions of the sulfonylureas currently on the U.S. market. All of the sulfonylureas listed below have generic alternatives.

• Chlorpropamide (Diabinese). This long-acting medication only requires once-a-day injection. Chlorpropamide is not recommended for the elderly or people with kidney disease, as it is eliminated slowly by the kidneys. Because this drug is long-acting, it may cause severe hypoglycemia, especially in the elderly.

• Glimepiride (Amaryl). This is the newest diabetes pill, introduced on the U.S. market in April 1996. Glimepiride is long acting and can be taken once a day. It has a very low risk of hypoglycemia and has less cardiac effect than any of the other sulfonylureas. This sulfonylurea has little impact on insulin release but appears to increase the action of existing insulin.

• Glipizide (Glucotrol, Glucotrol XL). Glipizide comes in two formulas: intermediate- and long-acting. It seems to be more effective when taken before meals. Caution should be used if taken by individuals with kidney or liver disease. This drug is the drug of choice for individuals starting therapy for Type II diabetes when diet and weight control have not been successful. Glipizide is well tolerated by the elderly.

• Glyburide (DiaBeta, Micronase, Glynase PresTab). This intermediate-acting drug should be taken once or twice a day. Even though it has intermediate action, the effects may last the entire day. Avoid use if you have liver or kidney problems. Glynase PresTab is the newest addition to this group and is more readily absorbed than the other preparations.

• Tolazamide (Ronase, Tolamide, Tolinase). Avoid using this intermediate-acting drug if you have severe kidney or liver disease. Usual dosing is once or twice daily.

• Tolbutamide (Orinase, Oramide). The short action of this drug reduces the risk of hypoglycemia. And because it is broken down completely by the liver, it leaves no active drug to pass through the kidneys and may be safe for individuals with kidney problems.

BIGUANIDES (by-GWAN-ides)

A new diabetes drug to the U.S. market is in the class biguanide. Called metformin (Glucophage), it has been used elsewhere around the world for about forty years. Rather than stimulate the pancreas, metformin lowers blood glucose levels by preventing the liver from releasing too much glucose. Therefore, because it doesn't increase insulin levels, it generally doesn't cause hypoglycemia. Other advantages to metformin are that some people lose weight when they start taking it, it reduces serum triglyceride levels, and improves the high-density/low-density lipoprotein ratio. For individuals who have not had good glucose control with sulfonylureas, metformin is a convenient drug to try. Side effects include a metallic taste in the mouth, diarrhea, and nausea.

ALPHA-GLUCOSIDASE INHIBITOR (al-fa glu-KAH-sid-ase)

Unlike sulfonylureas and metformin, acarbose (AK-er-bose), which entered the U.S. market in early 1996 under the trade name Precose, keeps blood glucose from rising so quickly after meals by delaying digestion of carbohydrates and absorption of glucose. This oral agent may be useful for people with Type I diabetes when taken along with their insulin. Side effects include flatulence, nausea, and diarrhea.

Choosing a Diabetes Pill

How do you decide which oral drug is best for you? You and your doctor will make that decision, based on your state of health and lifestyle. For example, if you have kidney problems, tolbutamide may be the drug of choice for you. However, if taking pills three times a day does not fit your lifestyle, you need to find another drug. If you are obese, metformin may be a better choice, as it is less likely to cause weight gain than a sulfonylurea.

Dosing and Side Effects

Diabetes pills are usually prescribed one type at a time. Occasionally, however, you may be taking the maximum recommended dose and still not be getting good glucose control. Rather than switch you to another drug, your doctor may combine two different medications. Combination therapy to be considered includes a sulfonylurea plus metformin; a sulfonylurea plus acarbose; or any one diabetes pill plus insulin.

Diabetes pills are usually taken with or before meals. If you forget to take your pills, do not "double up" at the next scheduled dosing time or change your schedule. Simply take your regular dose at your next prescribed time.

The most common side effect of diabetes pills is hypoglycemia. This is more likely to happen if you are taking a sulfonylurea than metformin. When you first start taking diabetes pills, you will need to monitor your blood glucose levels and pay careful attention to the timing of your meal, exercise, and dosing schedule. Keep your management team informed about any and all problems with your medication.

Other side effects of diabetes pills include loss of appetite, rashes, itching, and stomach and intestinal upset. In addition, if you are taking other medications or drink alcohol, you may experience adverse effects. Inform your doctor about all drugs you take, including nonprescription drugs and alcohol. Types of drugs known to cause adverse effects if taken along with diabetes pills include certain diuretics, birth control pills, estrogen supplements, and corticosteroids. Even aspirin, if taken in large amounts, can have an impact on how sulfonylureas work.

Glucagon

Glucagon is a hormone produced by the alpha cells in the pancreas. As a prescription medication, it is injected to treat hypoglycemia in semiconscious or unconscious people or in those who cannot or will not take food or liquids by mouth. Once injected, it triggers the glucose in the liver to enter the blood, thus raising the blood glucose level. We recommend you keep an emergency supply of glucagon in your home, car, and at work.

Medical Interventions for Diabetic Complications

Diligent blood glucose management, attention to overall health, and routine visits to your health-care team can significantly reduce or even eliminate the risk of developing some complications of diabetes. If serious complications do arise, medical intervention is usually required. Below we discuss some of the common diabetic complications and available treatments.

Kidney Damage (Nephropathy)

It is believed that good blood glucose control can reverse very early-stage proteinuria, but once kidney disease progresses past that stage, optimal blood glucose control can only help slow progression of the disease. There are no drugs to cure kidney disease, but your doctor may prescribe drugs to treat high blood pressure, which causes considerable damage to the kidneys. Drugs that help control high blood pressure are known as ACE (angiotensin converting enzyme) inhibitors (see "Hypertension," p. 235).

When 90 percent of kidney function is lost, dialysis—filtration of waste products from the blood—becomes necessary to stay alive. Two types of dialysis are available. In peritoneal dialysis, a minor surgical procedure is required, during which a plastic tube is inserted through your abdominal wall into the peritoneal cavity. This cavity has a membrane called the peritoneum, which acts as a filter through which your blood passes and is cleaned of waste products. The other type is hemodialysis, in which a tube is inserted into your arm and your blood flows out and is filtered through a device called a dialyzer. The dialyzer removes waste products from your blood and returns the clean blood to you.

Kidney transplantation is an option for individuals with end-stage renal failure, although it is not usually recommended for people older than sixty-five years. The best donors of kidneys are related family members, although success rates as high as 80 percent two years after transplantation are reported in people who receive kidneys from unrelated individuals. If you undergo kidney transplantation, you will need to take antirejection drugs for the rest of your life. If the transplanted kidney fails or your body rejects it, you will have the option to return to dialysis or receive another kidney. A newer approach to failed kidney transplantation is pancreas transplantation. Although this procedure is not widely performed, continued research and more transplants will hopefully make this option more available.

Retinopathy and Other Eye Problems

Problems that affect the retina of people with diabetes can be treated successfully using laser surgery. Laser surgery works best to prevent worsening of vision rather than to restore it, thus early detection of retinopathy and other eye problems is crucial.

In retinopathy, the tiny blood vessels, or capillaries, in the eye can become blocked and cause the blood vessels to leak. Blurred and double vision can result, with possible vision loss. Laser surgery burns and seals tiny areas of the leaking blood vessels and allows the retina to dry and function normally. The procedure takes a few minutes in the ophthalmologist's office, causes little, if any, discomfort, and can reduce risk of severe vision loss from diabetic retinopathy by 90 percent.

Sometimes abnormal retinal blood vessels bleed into the vitreous, the clear substance inside the eye. If this happens, you may see floating spots or have almost total loss of vision, depending on the amount of bleeding. Laser surgery can be performed once you allow much of the accumulated blood to be absorbed by the body.

Cataracts, when caught early, can often be reversed with good blood glucose control. When vision becomes significantly impaired, however, surgery is the only effective treatment available. Glaucoma responds to medication and laser surgery.

Neuropathy

When the nerves are damaged by chronic high blood glucose, it can cause moderate to severe pain in various parts of the body. To treat pain, your physician may prescribe aspirin or acetaminophen. To reduce nerve inflammation, nonsteroidal antiinflammatory drugs such as ibuprofen (e.g., Motrin, Advil) may be recommended. The antidepressant drugs promazine and amitriptyline, in lower dosages than given for depression, are often prescribed to relieve nerve irritation. Application of ointments that contain capsaicin (also see "Herbal Medicine" in Part II) is effective against pain when applied several times a day.

Newer drugs called aldose reductase inhibitors are being investigated as a means to block or reduce the effects of the chemical reactions that occur in people with diabetes and damage their nerves. Aldose reductase is an enzyme that is found in many parts of the body. Its role is to help change glucose into a sugar alcohol called sorbitol. If aldose reductase makes too much sorbitol, the sorbitol becomes trapped in the nerve cells and damages them, leading to neuropathy.

If the pain of neuropathy is chronic and severe, your physician may prescribe a TENS (transcutaneous electrical nerve stimulation) unit. A TENS device is a small power unit that delivers minute amounts of electrical current to a body site that is painful. It is a safe therapy and is especially helpful for people who have gotten little or no relief from medications. The TENS device is the size of a beeper and has wire leads with electrodes at the ends. The leads run under your clothing and the electrodes are placed on the treatment sites. A TENS unit must be prescribed by a physician.

Once the unit is turned on, a low level of electricity stimulates the nerve fibers and blocks the pain signals to the brain. Some experts say the electrical stimulation helps trigger the release of endorphins and enkaphalins—the body's natural pain relievers. The stimulation causes a slight tingling sensation for some people; others say they feel nothing at all. You can turn the unit on or off as needed.

During the early stages of therapy, 60 to 80 percent of chronic pain can be reduced. After about one year of use, however, only about 20 to 30 percent of TENS users continue to get relief.

TENS works best when you make it a *part* of your therapy. TENS can relieve pain, although it cannot prevent it. Natural therapies such as biofeedback and other relaxation techniques can help increase the effectiveness of TENS.

Hypertension

If diet and exercise have not been successful in lowering your high blood pressure to an acceptable level, your physician may prescribe blood pressure medication. Some of the most common drugs used for hypertension are diuretics (e.g., Dyazide, Diuril, Esidrix, and Maxzide), beta-blockers (e.g., Inderal, Lopressor, Tenormin, Visken), and calcium channel blockers (e.g., Calan, Adalat, Procardia), and ACE (angiotensin converting enzyme) inhibitors (e.g., Capoten, Lotensin, Vasotec, Zestril). However, it is important to carefully monitor your blood glucose levels as many of these drugs, especially diuretics and beta-blockers, can raise blood glucose levels. Drugs for hypertension should only be taken under supervision of your physician.

Summary

You have reached the end of this book, but not the end of the road. We hope we have opened up new avenues for you to explore and broadened your understanding not only of diabetes, but of some natural ways you can manage and control this disease.

Discoveries are being made every day in conventional medicine: new diabetes drugs, new uses for existing drugs, improved transplantation techniques, easier insulin delivery. At the same time, people like yourself are discovering the virtues of natural therapies, many of which are centuries old.

Most experts view diabetes as primarily a disease of lifestyle—the product of poor nutrition, lack of activity, obesity, high stress, and environmental toxins. Natural approaches can help heal all of these problems. For people who possess the desire and motivation, natural healing techniques have the potential to virtually eliminate the need for traditional medical therapy in people with Type II diabetes. Unfortunately, natural approaches cannot restore the production of insulin in people with Type I diabetes, although they can lessen their dependence on insulin.

In this book we have shown you that when it comes to your health, especially diabetes, you have choices. When you take a natural approach to treating diabetes and its complications, you establish a dialogue with your body. Diabetes is one condition in which the mind/body dialogue is critical, for open communication can allow you to participate more fully in management of the disease: to ward off episodes of hypoglycemia and hyperglycemia and, in the longer view, complications associated with diabetes. When you make natural healing approaches a part of your life, you reap the benefits of better control of diabetes and of your life.

And that can make you feel good.

Feel good.

GLOSSARY

ACE Inhibitor: Type of drug used to lower blood pressure. It may also help prevent or slow the progression of kidney disease in people with diabetes.

Acute: Something that happens for a limited period of time and/or that comes on abruptly.

Adrenal Glands: Two organs that sit on top of the kidneys and make and release hormones such as adrenaline (epinephrine).

Albuminuria: An excess amount of protein called albumin in the urine. Albuminuria may indicate kidney disease.

Aldose Reductase Inhibitor: A class of drugs under investigation as a way to prevent eye and nerve damage in people with diabetes.

Alpha Cell: A type of cell in the pancreas that makes and releases the hormone glucagon.

Angiopathy: A disease of the blood vessels (arteries, veins, and capillaries) that occurs when someone has diabetes for a long time.

Antigens: Substances that cause an immune response in the body. The body perceives the antigens to be harmful and thus produces antibodies to attack and destroy the antigens.

Arteriosclerosis: A group of diseases in which the artery walls get thick and hard, slowing blood flow.

Artery: A large blood vessel that carries blood from the heart to other parts of the body.

Atherosclerosis: One of many diseases in which fat builds up in the large- and medium-sized arteries.

Beta Cell: A type of cell in the pancreas that makes and releases insulin, a hormone that controls the blood glucose level.

Blood Glucose: The main sugar the body makes from food, especially carbohydrates. Glucose is the major energy source for cells.

Blood Glucose Meter: A machine that helps measure the amount of glucose in the blood.

Blood Pressure: The force of the blood on the artery walls.

Blood Urea Nitrogen (BUN): Waste product produced by the kidneys. Raised BUN levels in the blood may indicate early kidney damage.

Capillary: The smallest blood vessels in the body.

Capsaicin: An ointment made from chili peppers used to relieve the pain of peripheral neuropathy.

Carbohydrate: One of the three main classes of foods. They are an energy source and consist mainly of starches and sugars.

Cataract: Clouding of the lens of the eye.

Cholesterol: A fatlike substance found in blood, muscle, liver, and other human and animal tissues. Excess cholesterol in the arteries can cause heart disease.

Chronic: Something that lasts a long time. Diabetes is an example of chronic disease.

Creatinine: A chemical in the blood that is eliminated through urine. A test of the amount of creatinine in the blood and/or urine indicates if the kidneys are working right.

Diabetes Control and Complications Trial (DCCT): A ten-year study (1983–1993) funded by the National Institute of Diabetes and Digestive and Kidney Diseases which assessed the effects of intensive therapy on the long-term complications of diabetes.

Diabetes Mellitus: A disease that occurs when the body cannot use insulin adequately or has none of its own to use.

Diabetic Ketoacidosis: Severe hyperglycemia that requires emergency treatment.

Diabetic Retinopathy: A disease of the capillaries of the retina of the eye.

Dialysis: A method that removes waste products such as urea from the blood when the kidneys can no longer perform this function. There are two types of dialysis: hemodialysis and peritoneal.

Diuretic: A drug that increases the flow of urine to help eliminate extra fluid from the body.

Endocrine Glands: Glands that release hormones into the bloodstream and impact metabolism.

End-Stage Renal Disease (ESRD): The final phase of kidney disease.

Epinephrine: Also called adrenaline, it is secreted by the adrenal glands and helps the liver release glucose.

Exchange Lists: Foods grouped according to type, which helps people with diabetes determine their eating plan.

Fasting Blood Glucose Test: A technique that determines how much glucose is in the blood. The normal range for blood glucose in people without diabetes is 70 to 110 mg/dL; levels higher than 140 mg/dL usually indicate diabetes.

Fats: One of the three main classes of foods and a source of energy in the body.

Fiber: Substance in food plants that helps the digestive process, lowers cholesterol, and helps control blood glucose levels.

Gangrene: Dead body tissue, usually caused by loss of blood flow.

Gastroparesis: A form of nerve damage that affects the stomach.

Gestational Diabetes Mellitus: A type of diabetes that can occur when a woman is pregnant. It usually resolves after the birth.

Glaucoma: An eye disease characterized by increased pressure in the eye.

Glomeruli: Tiny blood vessels in the kidneys where the blood is filtered and waste products are eliminated.

Glucagon: A hormone made in the pancreas that raises the level of glucose in the blood.

Glucose: A simple sugar found in the blood that is the body's main source of energy. See also: Blood glucose.

Glucose Tolerance Test (GTT): A test that shows how well the body deals with glucose in the blood over time; used to see if a person has diabetes. A first blood sample is taken in the morning before the person has eaten; then the person drinks a liquid that has glucose in it. After one hour, a second blood sample is taken and then, one hour later, a third.

Glycogen: A substance composed of sugars that is stored in the liver and muscles and releases glucose into the blood when needed by cells.

Glycosylated Hemoglobin Test: A blood test that measures a person's average blood glucose for the two- to three-month period before the test.

Hemodialysis: A mechanical way to remove waste products from the blood. See also: Dialysis.

Hemoglobin: The substance in red blood cells that carries oxygen to the cells.

High Blood Pressure: When blood flows through the vessels at a greater than normal force.

Hormone: A chemical released by special cells that "tells" other cells what to do.

Human Insulin: Man-made insulins that are similar to insulin produced by the human body.

Hyperglycemia: Glucose level that is too high in the blood.

Hypertension: Blood pressure that is above normal. See also: High blood pressure.

Hypoglycemia: Glucose level that is too low in the blood.

Impaired Glucose Tolerance (IGT): Blood glucose levels that are higher than normal but not so high as to be considered diabetes.

Implantable Insulin Pump: A small pump placed inside of the body that delivers insulin on demand from a handheld programmer.

Impotence: The inability to attain and maintain an erect penis and to emit semen.

Insulin: A hormone produced in the pancreas that helps the body use glucose for energy.

Insulin-Dependent Diabetes Mellitus: A chronic condition in which the pancreas makes little or no insulin because the beta cells have been destroyed. Also called Type I diabetes.

Insulin Pump: A beeper-size device that delivers a continuous supply of insulin into the body.

Insulin Reaction: A response to a too-low level of glucose in the blood; also called hypoglycemia.

Insulin Receptors: Sites on the outer part of a cell that allow the cell to join with insulin.

Insulin Resistance: When the body produces insulin but is unable to respond properly to it.

Intensive Therapy: A method of treatment for Type I diabetes in which the goal is to keep blood glucose levels as close to normal as possible. Also recommended for Type II diabetes.

Jet Injector: A device that uses high pressure to delivery insulin through the skin and into the body.

Ketoacidosis: See Diabetic ketoacidosis.

Ketones: Chemicals the body makes when there is insufficient insulin in the blood and it must break down fat for its energy.

Ketosis: A condition in which ketone bodies build up in body tissues and fluids. Ketosis can lead to ketoacidosis.

Kidney Disease: Also called nephropathy, kidney disease can be any one of several chronic conditions that are caused by damage to the cells of the kidney.

Kidneys: Two organs in the lower back that clean waste and poisons from the blood.

Lente Insulin: An intermediate-acting insulin.

Metformin: Drug used to treat Type II diabetes; in the drug class called biguanides.

Nephropathy: Kidney diseases caused by damage to the small blood vessels or to the units in the kidneys that filter the blood.

Neuropathy: Disease of the nervous system. See also: Peripheral neuropathy.

Non–Insulin-Dependent Diabetes Mellitus (NIDDM): Also called Type II diabetes; most common form of diabetes mellitus. People with NIDDM produce some insulin but the body cannot use it properly.

NPH Insulin: An intermediate-acting insulin.

Obesity: When people have 20 percent or more extra body fat for their age, height, sex, and bone structure.

Oral Glucose Tolerance Test (OGTT): A test to see if a person has diabetes. See: Glucose tolerance test.

Pancreas: An organ behind the lower part of the stomach that makes insulin and enzymes that help the body digest food.

Peripheral Neuropathy: Nerve damage that usually affects the feet and legs.

Peritoneal Dialysis: A mechanical way to clean the blood of people with kidney disease.

Polydipsia: Great thirst that lasts for long periods of time.

Polyphagia: Great hunger.

Polyunsaturated Fats: Fat that comes from vegetables.

Polyuria: A need to urinate often.

Protein: One of the three main classes of food. Proteins are found in many foods, including soy products, beans, legumes, vegetables, and animal products.

Proteinuria: Presence of too much protein in the urine; may signal kidney damage.

Regular Insulin: A fast-acting insulin.

Retina: Center part of the back lining of the eye that senses light.

Retinopathy: A disease of the small blood vessels in the retina of the eye. See also: Diabetic retinopathy.

Saturated Fat: A type of fat that comes primarily from animals.

Secondary Diabetes: Diabetes that develops because of another disease or because of taking certain drugs or chemicals.

Sorbitol: The body produces this sugar alcohol which, if levels get too high, may cause damage to the eyes and nerves.

Sucrose: Table sugar; a form of sugar the body must break down into a simpler form before the blood can use it.

Sulfonylureas: Pills that lower the level of glucose in the blood.

Syringe: A device used to inject medications or other liquids into body tissues. An insulin syringe has a hollow plastic or glass tube with a plunger inside. The plunger forces the insulin through the needle into the body.

Tolazamide: A pill that lowers the level of glucose in the blood.

Tolbutamide: A pill that lowers the level of glucose in the blood.

Transcutaneous Electronic Nerve Stimulation (TENS): A treatment for painful neuropathy.

Trigylceride: A type of blood fat.

Type I Diabetes Mellitus: Insulin-dependent diabetes mellitus.

Type II Diabetes Mellitus: Non–insulin-dependent diabetes mellitus.

U-100: A unit of insulin. Means one hundred units of insulin per milliliter or cubic centimeter of solution.

Ulcer: A break in the skin or deep sore. People with diabetes often get ulcers caused by minor scrapes on the feet or legs.

Ultralente Insulin: A long-acting insulin.

Urea: One of the main waste products of the body. The kidneys flush urea away in the urine.

Urine Testing: Test of urine to see if it contains glucose and ketones.

Information and Products by Topic

Contact the following organizations for referrals and general information. Those without a phone listing prefer written inquiries. When writing for information, please send a business-size self-addressed stamped envelope.

Diabetes: General Information

American Association of Diabetes Educators
 444 North Michigan Avenue, Suite 1240
 Chicago, IL 60611-3901
 (312) 644-2233 or 1-800-338-3633
 Continuing education programs and a certification program for diabetes educators; publishes a monthly journal and other resources.

American Diabetes Association (ADA)
 1660 Duke Street
 P.O. Box 25757
 Alexandria, VA 22313
 (800) 232-3472 or (703) 549-1500
 Publishes bimonthly magazine, *Diabetes Forecast*. Fosters public awareness of diabetes and supports and promotes diabetes research and education. Local affiliates are listed in telephone directories or can be located by contacting the national office.

The American Dietetic Association, National Center for Nutrition and Dietetics
216 West Jackson Boulevard
Chicago, IL 60606-6995
(800) 366-1655 or (312) 899-0040
Professional organization for registered dietitians. Publishes materials for patient and professional education and runs an information and referral service for the general public.

Centers for Disease Control (CDC), National Center for Chronic Disease Prevention and Health Promotion
4770 Buford Highway
The Rhodes Building, MS K-13
Atlanta, GA 30341-3724
Technical Information Services Branch
(770) 488-5080
Agency of the Federal Government that has information on the surveillance and prevention of diabetes for health-care professionals and people with diabetes.

International Diabetes Center
3800 Park Nicollet Boulevard
Minneapolis, MN 55416
(612) 993-3393
Offers pamphlets, booklets, and slide sets.

Joslin Diabetes Center
One Joslin Place
Boston, MA 02215
(617) 732-2400
World-famous foundation with divisions for research, education, and youth.

Juvenile Diabetes Foundation (JDF) International
120 Wall Street, 19th Floor
New York, NY 10005
(800) 223-1138 or (212) 889-7575
Private, voluntary organization that promotes research and public education in diabetes, primarily Type I. Local chapters are listed in telephone directories or can be found by contacting the national office.

National Diabetes Information Clearinghouse
1 Information Way
Bethesda, MD 20892-3560
(301) 654-3327
A service of NIDDK. Distributes diabetes-related materials to the public and to health professionals.

National Eye Health Education Program
National Eye Institute
National Institutes of Health, Box 20/20
Bethesda, MD 20892
(301) 496-5248

National Heart, Lung, and Blood Institute
2366 Eastlake Avenue E., Suite 322
Seattle, WA 98102
(206) 323-7610

Natural Healing: General Information

American Association of Naturopathic Physicians
P.O. Box 2579
Kirkland, WA 98083-2579
(206) 827-6035

American Holistic Health Association
P.O. Box 17400
Anaheim, CA 92817-7400
(714) 779-6152

The American Institute of Stress
124 Park Avenue
Yonkers, NY 10703
(800) 24-RELAX
Information about mind/body relationships and stress in health. Publishes a monthly newsletter available to the public.

Complementary Medicine Association
4649 East Malvern Street
Tucson, AZ 85711
(602) 323-6291
Networking and referral service.

Office of Alternative Medicine/National Institutes of Health
9000 Rockville Pike, Building 31, Room 5B-38
Bethesda, MD 20892
(301) 402-2466

Acupressure and Acupuncture

American Academy of Medical Acupuncture
5820 Wilshire Boulevard, Suite 500
Los Angeles, CA 90036
(213) 937-5514

American Association of Acupuncture and Oriental Medicine
433 Front Street
Catasauqua, PA 18032
(610) 433-2448

American Oriental Bodywork Association
Glendale Executive Campus
1000 White Horse Road, Suite 510
Voorhees, NJ 08043
(609) 782-1616

Biofeedback

Biofeedback Certification Institute of America
10200 West 44th Avenue, Suite 304
Wheatridge, CO 80033-2840
(303) 420-2902

Life Sciences Institute of Mind/Body Health
2955 SW Wanamaker Drive, Suite B
Topeka, KS 66614
(913) 271-8686

Gerson Therapy

Gerson Institute and Cancer Curing Society
P.O. Box 430
Bonita, CA 91908
(888) 4-GERSON or (619) 585-7600

Herbal Medicine

American Botanical Council
  P.O. Box 201660
  Austin, TX 78720-1660
  (800) 373-7105 or (512) 331-8868

Herb Society of America
  9019 Kirtland Chardon Road
  Kirtland, OH 44094
  (216) 256-0514

Homeopathic

Homeopathic Academy of Naturopathic Physicians
  12132 SE Foster Place
  Portland, OR 97266
  (503) 761-3298

Homeopathic Educational Services
  2124 Kittredge Street
  Berkeley, CA 94704
  (510) 649-0294

International Foundation for Homeopathy
  P.O. Box 7
  Edmonds, WA 98020
  (206) 776-4147

National Center for Homeopathy
  801 N. Fairfax Street, Suite 306
  Alexandria, VA 22314
  (703) 548-7790

Hypnosis

Society for Clinical and Experimental Hypnosis
  3905 Vincennes Road, Suite 304
  Indianapolis, IN 46268
  (317) 872-7093
  (847) 297-3317
  Please send SASE for information.

Massage

American Massage Therapy Association
  820 Davis Street, Suite 100
  Evanston, IL 60601-4444
  (312) 761-AMTA

Nutrition

Linus Pauling Institute
  Oregon State University
  571 Weniger Hall
  Corvallis, OR 97331-6512
  (541) 737-5075 (for vitamin therapy information)

The McDougall Program
  P.O. Box 14039
  Santa Rosa, CA 95402
  (707) 576-1654

North American Vegetarian Society
  P.O. Box 72
  Dolgeville, NY 13329
  (518) 568-7970

Physicians Committee for Responsible Medicine
  P.O. Box 6322
  Washington DC 20015
  (202) 686-2210

Oxygen Therapy

The American College of Hyperbaric Medicine
  Ocean Medical Center
  4001 Ocean Drive, Suite 303
  Lauderdale-by-the-Sea, FL 33308
  (954) 771-4000

International Bio-Oxidative Medicine Foundation
  P.O. Box 891954
  Oklahoma City, OK 73189
  (405) 478-IBOM

The Undersea and Hyperbaric Medical Society
  10531 Metropolitan Avenue
  Kensington, MD 20895
  (301) 942-2980

Polarity Therapy

American Polarity Therapy Association
  2888 Bluff Street, Suite 149
  Boulder, CO 80301
  (303) 545-2080

Reflexology

International Institute of Reflexology
  P.O. Box 12642
  St. Petersburg, FL 33733-2642
  (813) 343-4811

Tai Chi

Complementary Medicine Association
  4649 East Malvern Street
  Tucson, AZ 85711
  (520) 323-6291

Visualization

The Academy for Guided Imagery
  P.O. Box 2070
  Mill Valley, CA 94942
  (800) 726-2070
  For guided imagery workshops and seminars.

Center for Spiritual Awareness
  P.O. Box 7
  Lake Rabun Road
  Lakemont, GA 30552
  (706) 782-4723

The Institute of Transpersonal Psychology
744 San Antonio Road
Palo Alto, CA 94303
(415) 493-4430
Imagery training; mind/body consciousness and wellness
workshops.

Yoga

International Association of Yoga Therapists
20 Sunnyside Avenue #A243
Mill Valley, CA 94941
(415) 868-2524

APPENDIX B

Sources for Herbs, Homeopathic Remedies, Audiovisuals

Herbs

East Earth Herb Inc.
  P.O. Box 2802
  Eugene, OR 97402
  (800) 827-HERB

Jean's Greens
  RR 1, Box 55J
  Rensselaerville, NY 12147
  (518) 239-8327

Mountain Herbal
  112 Main Street
  Montpelier, VT 05602
  (802) 223-0888

Mountain Rose Herbs
  P.O. Box 2000
  Redway, CA 95560
  (707) 923-3941

Nature's Way
  10 Mountain Springs Parkway
  Springville, UT 84663
  Available in stores.

OSO Herbals
  P.O. Box 50306-278
  Tucson, AZ 85703
  (520) 624-9225

Terra Firma Botanicals
  P.O. Box 5680
  Eugene, OR 97405
  (541) 485-7726
  Fresh and dried herbal extracts; massage oils; $1 catalog.

Homeopathy

Boericke & Tafel, Inc.
  2381 Circadian Way
  Santa Rosa, CA 95407
  Available in stores.

Homeopathy Overnight
  RR 1, Box 818
  Kingfield, ME 04947
  (800) ARNICA30
  Mail-order homeopathic remedies.

Homeopathic Educational Services
  2124 Kittredge Street
  Berkeley, CA 94704
  (510) 649-0294 information; (800) 359-9051 orders only
  Comprehensive catalog of remedies, books, tapes, and cassettes.

Massage

Massage Magazine
  1315 West Mallon Street
  Spokane, WA 99201
  (509) 324-8117
  Bimonthly; massage, bodywork, and related healing arts.

Meditation/Visualization Tapes

The BodyMind Audio Tape Program
  Jeanne Achterberg, PhD
  New Era Media/The Arc Group

P.O. Box 410685-BT
San Francisco, CA 94141
(415) 863-3555
Audiotapes for diabetes, hypertension, general relaxation,
pain, weight loss, immune system enhancement.

Image Paths, Inc.
2635 Payne Avenue
Cleveland, OH 44114
(800) 800-8661
The audiotape series called *Health Journeys* has guided imagery tapes for diabetes, high blood pressure, heart disease,
depression, pain, and many other conditions.

Mind/Body Health Sciences, Inc.
393 Dixon Road
Boulder, CO 80302-7177
(303) 440-8460
Relaxation cassettes and videos by the Joan and Miroslav
Borysenko.

QuantumQuests
P.O. Box 98
Oakview, CA 93022
(800) 772-0090

The Source Cassette Learning System
Emmet Miller, MD
770 Menlo Avenue, #200
Menlo Park, CA 94025
(415) 328-7171
Tapes for relaxation, pain relief. Free catalog.

Nutrition

The Nutrition Action Health Letter
Center for Science in the Public Interest
1875 Connecticut Avenue, NW, Suite 300
Washington, D.C. 20009-5728
(202) 332-9111
Monthly newsletter for the general public.

Vegetarian Journal
  Vegetarian Resource Group
  P.O. Box 1463
  Baltimore, MD 21203
  (410) 366-8343

Vegetarian Voice
  North American Vegetarian Society
  P.O. Box 72
  Dolgeville, NY 13329
  (518) 568-7970
  Focus: health, compassionate living, and environment; recipes.

Vegetarian Times
  P.O. Box 570
  Oak Park, IL 60303
  (708) 848-8100
  Monthly publication; articles on health, nutrition, and cooking.

Yoga

Himalayan Institute of Yoga, Science and Philosophy
  RR 1, Box 400
  Honesdale, PA 18431
  (717) 253-5551
  Catalog; also publishes the magazine *Yoga International*.

Samata Yoga and Health Institute
  4150 Tivoli Avenue
  Los Angeles, CA 90066
  (310) 306-8845
  Manuals, videos, and audio cassettes; also offers classes.

Total Yoga (video)
  White Lotus Foundation
  2500 San Marcos Pass
  Santa Barbara, CA 93105
  (805) 964-1944

Bibliography and Suggested Reading

Diabetes

Bennion, Lynn J. "Hypoglycemia: A Diagnostic Challenge," *Clinical Diabetes* (July/August 1985): 85–90.

DCCT Research Group. "Epidemiology of Severe Hypoglycemia in the Diabetes Control and Complications Trial." *The American Journal of Medicine* 90 (April 1991): 450–459.

Field, James B. "Hypoglycemia: Definition, Clinical Presentations, Classifications and Laboratory Tests." In *Endocrinology and Metabolism Clinics of North America* 18, no. 1 (March 1989).

Foster, Daniel, and Arthur Rubenstein. "Hypoglycemia, Insulinoma, and Other Hormone-Secreting Tumors of the Pancreas." In *Principles of Internal Medicine,* ed. E. Braunwald et al. New York: McGraw-Hill Book Company, 1987.

Franz, Marion, et al. *Learning to Live Well with Diabetes.* Minneapolis: DCI Publishing, 1991.

Helgason T., and M. R. Johasson. "Evidence for a Food Additive as a Cause of Ketosis-Prone Diabetes." *Lancet* 88 (1981): 716–720.

Leslie C. A., et al. Psychological insulin resistance: a missed diagnosis? *Diabetes Spectrum* 7 (1994): 52–57.

Lowe, Ernest, and Gary Arsham. *Diabetes: A Guide to Living Well.* Wayzuta, MN: Diabetes Center, Inc., 1989.

Milchovich, Sue, and Barbara Dunn-Long. *Diabetes Mellitus: A Practical Handbook*. Menlo Park: Bull Publishing, 1990.

Rayfield, Elliot J., M.D., and Cheryl Solimini. *Diabetes: Beating the Odds: The Doctor's Guide to Reducing Your Risk*. Reading, Mass.: Addison-Wesley, 1992.

Raymond, Mike. *The Human Side of Diabetes*. Chicago: Noble Press, 1992.

Service, F. John. "Hypoglycemic Disorders." *New England Journal of Medicine* (27 April 1995): 1,144–1,152.

Time. "What Triggers Diabetes? Compelling New Evidence Suggests a Viral Infection Could Be the Culprit." 144, no. 14 (3 October 1994).

Whitaker, Julian, M.D. *Reversing Diabetes*. New York: Warner Books, 1987.

Acupressure and Acupuncture

Bauer, Cathryn. *Acupressure for Everyone*. New York: Henry Holt, 1991.

Cargill, Marie. *Acupuncture: A Viable Medical Alternative*. Westport, Conn.: Praeger, 1994.

Gach, Michael Reed. *Acupressure's Potent Points: A Guide to Self-Care for Common Ailments*. New York: Bantam, 1990.

Houston, F. M. *The Healing Benefits of Acupressure*. Rev. ed. New Canaan, Conn.: Keats, 1994.

Kaptchuk, Ted. *The Web That Has No Weaver: Understanding Chinese Medicine*. New York: Congdon & Weed, 1993.

Kenyon, Keith, M.D. *Pressure Points: Do-It-Yourself Acupuncture Without Needles*. New York: Arco, 1984.

Lundberg, Paul. *The Book of Shiatsu*. London: Gaia Books, 1992.

Marcus, Paul. *Acupuncture: A Patient's Guide*. New York: Thorsons, 1985.

———. *Thorsons Introductory Guide to Acupuncture*. London: Hammersmith, 1991.

Nickel, David J. *Acupressure for Athletes*. New York: Henry Holt, 1987.

Ohashi, Wataru. *Do-It-Yourself Shiatsu*. New York: Viking, 1992.

Serizawa, Katsusuke, M.D. *Tsubo: Vital Points for Oriental Therapy*. Tokyo: Japan Publications, 1976.

Stux, Gabriel. *Basics of Acupuncture*. Berlin, New York: Springer-Verlag, 1988.

Thompson, Gerry. *The Shiatsu Manual*. New York: Sterling Publishing, 1994.

Biofeedback

Green, Elmer. *Beyond Biofeedback*. New York: Delacorte, 1977.
Sedlacek, Kurt. *The Sedlacek Technique: Finding the Calm*. New York: McGraw-Hill, 1989.

Herbal Medicine

Carroll, David. *The Complete Book of Natural Medicine*. New York: Summit Books, 1980.
Castleman, Michael. *The Healing Herbs*. Emmaus, PA: Rodale Press, 1991.
Elias, Jason, and Shelagh Masline. *Healing Herbal Remedies*. New York: Dell, 1995.
Hoffman, David. *The New Holistic Herbal*. Rockport, MA: Element Books, 1992.
Inglis, Brian, and Ruth West. *The Alternative Health Guide*. New York: Knopf, 1983.
Kloss, Jethro. *Back to Eden*. Rev. ed. Loma Linda, CA: Back to Eden Books Publishing Co., 1994.
Lucas, Richard M. *Miracle Medicine Herbs*. Englewood Cliffs, NJ: Prentice-Hall, 1990.
Mayell, Mark. *Off-the-Shelf Natural Health: How to Use Herbs and Nutrients to Stay Well*. New York: Bantam Books, 1995.
Mills, Simon, and Steven Finando. *Alternatives in Healing*. New York: NAL Books, 1989.
Mindell, Earl, R.Ph., Ph.D. *Earl Mindell's Herb Bible*. New York: Simon & Schuster, 1992.
Moore, Michael. *Medicinal Plants of the Desert and Canyon West*. Santa Fe, NM: Museum of New Mexico Press, 1989.
Murray, Michael T., N.D. *The Healing Power of Herbs*. Rocklin, Cal.: Prima Publishing, 1991.
———. *Natural Alternatives to Over-the-Counter and Prescription Drugs*. New York: Morrow, 1994.
Ody, Penelope. *The Complete Medicinal Herbal*. New York: Dorling Kindersley, 1993.
Shanmugasundaram, E.R.B., et al: "Use of *Gymnema sylvestre* Leaf Extract in the Control of Blood Glucose in Insulin-Dependent Diabetes Mellitus. *J Ethnopharmacol* 30 (1990): 281–294.

Sherman, John A., N.D. *The Complete Botanical Prescriber.* Compiled by John A. Sherman, 1993.

Stein, Diane. *All Women Are Healers.* Freedom, CA.: The Crossing Press, 1990.

Tierra, Lesley. *The Herbs of Life: Health and Healing Using Western and Chinese Techniques.* Freedom, CA.: The Crossing Press, 1992.

Tierra, Michael, N.D. *Planetary Herbology.* Twin Lakes, Wis.: Lotus Press, 1988.

———. *The Way of Herbs.* New York: Simon & Schuster, 1990.

Trattler, Ross. *Better Health Through Natural Healing.* New York: McGraw-Hill, 1985.

Tyler, Varro E., *The Honest Herbal.* 3rd ed. Binghamton, NY: Haworth Press, 1993.

Homeopathy

Blackie, Margery G. *The Patient Not the Cure: The Challenge of Homeopathy.* Santa Barbara, Cal.: Westbridge Press, 1978.

Coulter, C. *Portraits of Homeopathic Medicine.* 2 vols. Berkeley: North Atlantic Books, 1986.

Cummings, Stephen, and Dana Ullman. *Everybody's Guide to Homeopathic Medicine.* Los Angeles: Jeremy P. Tarcher, 1991.

Gibson, D. M. *Studies of Homeopathic Remedies.* Beaconsfield, England: Beaconsfield Publishers, 1987.

Grossinger, Richard. *Homeopathy: An Introduction for Skeptics and Beginners.* Berkeley, Cal.: North Atlantic Books, 1993.

Hahnemann, Samuel. *The Organon of Medicine.* Translated by J. Kunli, A. Naude, and P. Pendleton. London: Gollancz, 1986.

Hammond, Christopher. *How to Use Homeopathy Effectively.* Nottingham, England, 1988.

Koehler, Gerhard. *The Handbook of Homeopathy.* Wellingborough, England, and New York: Thorsons, 1986.

Lessell, Dr. Colin B. *The World Travellers' Manual of Homeopathy.* Essex, England: C. W. Daniel Company, Ltd., 1993.

Lockie, Andrew. *The Home Guide to Homeopathy.* New York: Simon & Schuster, 1989; 1993.

Mills, Simon, and Steven J. Finando. *Alternatives in Healing.* New York: New American Library, 1988.

Panos, Maesimund B. *Homeopathic Medicine at Home.* Los Angeles: Jeremy P. Tarcher, 1980.

Rose, Barry. *The Family Health Guide to Homeopathy.* Berkeley: Celestial Arts, 1992.

Stephenson, James H. *A Doctor's Guide to Helping Yourself with Homeopathic Remedies.* 1st British ed. Wellingborough, England: Thorsons, 1977.

Ullman, Dana. *Homeopathy: Medicine for the 21st Century.* Berkeley: North Atlantic Books, 1988.

———. *Discovering Homeopathy.* Berkeley: North Atlantic Books, 1991.

Weiner, Michael. *The Complete Book of Homeopathy.* Garden City, NY: Avery Publishing Group, 1989.

Weinstein, Corey, and Nancy Bruning. *Healing Homeopathic Remedies.* New York: Dell, 1996.

Hypnosis

Alman, Brian M. *Self-Hypnosis: The Complete Manual.* New York: Brunner/Mazel, 1992.

Copelan, Rachael. *How to Hypnotize Yourself and Others.* New York: Bell Publishing, 1984.

Fisher, Stanley. *Discovering the Power of Self-Hypnosis.* New York: HarperCollins, 1991.

Haley, Jay. *Uncommon Therapy.* New York: Norton, 1987.

Hilgad, Ernest. *Hypnosis: In the Relief of Pain.* New York: Brunner/Mazel, 1994.

Miller, Michael M.D. *Therapeutic Hypnosis.* New York: Human Sciences Press, 1979.

Wallace, Benjamin. *Applied Hypnosis.* Chicago: Nelson-Hall, 1979.

Yates, John. *The Complete Book of Self-Hypnosis.* Chicago: Nelson-Hall, 1984.

Massage

Anhui Medical School, China. *Chinese Massage.* Point Roberts, WA: Hartley & Marks, 1987.

DePaoli, Carlo. *The Healing Touch of Massage.* New York: Sterling, 1995.

Inkeles, Gordon. *The Art of Sensual Massage.* New York: Simon & Schuster, 1974.

Kaptchuk, Ted. *The Web That Has No Weaver. Understanding Chinese Medicine.* New York: Congdon & Weed, 1993.

Kushi, Michio, and Edward Esko, *Basic Shiatsu*. Becket, MA: One Peaceful World Press, 1995.

Lidell, Lucinda, et al. *The Book of Massage*. New York: Simon & Schuster, 1984.

Ravald, Bertild. *The Art of Swedish Massage*. New York: Dutton, 1984.

Tappan, Frances M. *Healing Massage Techniques*. Stamford, CT: Appleton & Lange, 1988.

Medical/Drug Therapies

Cooney, Gerard, et al., ed. *The American Druggist's Complete Family Guide to Prescriptions, Pills, and Drugs*. New York: Hearst Books, 1995.

Ford, E. S., and W. H. Herman "Leisure-Time Physical Activity Patterns in the U.S. Diabetic Population. Findings from the 1990 National Health Interview Survey—Health Promotion and Disease Prevention Supplement." *Diabetes Care* 18(1) (January 1995): 27–33.

Griffith, H. Winter, M.D. *Complete Guide to Prescription and Non-Prescription Drugs, 1995 ed*. New York: Berkley Publishing Group, 1994.

Long, James W., MD. *The Essential Guide to Prescription Drugs*. New York: HarperPerennial, 1995.

Monthly Prescribing Reference. New York: Prescribing Reference, January 1995.

1996 Physicians GenRx. St. Louis: Mosby Year Book, 1996.

Schein, Jeffrey, and Philip Hansten. *Consumer's Guide to Drug Interactions*. New York: Collier Books, 1993.

United States Pharmacopeial Convention, Inc. *About Your Medicines*. Rockville, MD: United States Pharmacopeial Convention, 1993.

West Georgia Center for Metabolic Disorders. *The Metabolic Page*. Columbia Doctors Hospital, Columbus, GA.

Winter, Ruth. *Consumer's Dictionary of Medicines*. New York: Crown, 1993.

Meditation, Visualization/Imagery

Borysenko, Joan. *Minding the Body, Mending the Mind*. Toronto/New York: Bantam Books, 1988.

————. *The Power of the Mind to Heal.* Carson, CA: Hay House, 1994.

Dunham, Eileen, and Cindy Cooper. *Therapeutic Relaxation and Imagery Development Manual.* Cupertino, CA: Health Horizons, 1989.

Epstein, Gerald. *Healing Visualizations.* New York: Bantam Books, 1989.

Fanning, Patrick. *Visualization for Change.* Oakland: New Harbinger, 1988.

Fezler, William. *Creative Imagery.* New York: Simon & Schuster, 1989.

Lusk, Julie, ed. *30 Scripts for Relaxation, Imagery and Inner Healing.* 2 vols. Duluth: Whole Person Associates, 1992.

McDonald, Kathleen. *How to Meditate.* Boston: Wisdom Publications, 1992.

Moen, Larry, ed. *Guided Imagery.* 2 vols. Naples: United States Publishing, 1992.

Naparstek, Belleruth. *Staying Well with Guided Imagery.* New York: Time Warner, 1994.

Ornstein, Robert, and David Sobel. *The Healing Mind.* New York: Simon & Schuster, 1987.

Pelletier, Kenneth R. *Mind as Healer, Mind as Slayer.* Rev. ed. New York: Delacorte, 1992.

Rossman, Martin L., M.D. *Healing Yourself: A Step-by-Step Program for Better Health Through Imagery.* New York: Walker & Co., 1987.

Samuels, Michael, M.D. *Healing with the Mind's Eye: A Guide for Using Imagery and Visions for Personal Growth and Healing.* New York: Simon & Schuster, 1990.

Siegel, Bernie S., M.D. *Peace, Love & Healing: Bodymind Communication and the Path to Self-Healing.* New York: Harper & Row, 1989.

Movement Therapy

Cantu, Robert C., M.D. *Diabetes and Exercise.* New York: Dutton, 1982.

Natural Medicine/Holistic Health

The Burton Goldberg Group. *Alternative Medicine: The Definitive Guide.* Puyallup, Wash.: Futura Medicine Publishing, 1994.

Chopra, Deepak, M.D. *Perfect Health: The Complete Mind/Body Guide.* New York: Harmony Books, 1991.

————. *Quantum Healing: Exploring the Frontiers of Body, Mind, Medicine.* New York: Bantam Books, 1993.

Cousins, Norman. *Anatomy of an Illness as Perceived by the Patient.* New York: Norton, 1979.

————. *Head First: The Biology of Hope and the Healing Power of the Human Spirit.* New York: Viking, 1990.

Dienstfrey, Harris. *Where the Mind Meets the Body.* New York: HarperCollins, 1991.

Frahm, David and Anna. *Reclaim Your Health.* Colorado Springs, CO: Pinon Press, 1995.

Goleman, Daniel, and Joel Gurin. *Mind Body Medicine: How to Use Your Mind for Better Health.* Yonkers, NY: Consumer Reports Books, 1993.

Kabat-Zinn, Jon. *Full Catastrophic Living: Using the Wisdom of Your Body and Mind to Face Stress, Pain, and Illness.* New York: Delacorte, 1990.

Marti, James. *The Alternative Health and Medicine Encyclopedia.* Detroit: Visible Ink Press, 1995.

Monte, Tom, et al. *World Medicine: The East-West Guide to Healing Your Body.* New York: Jeremy P. Tarcher, 1993.

Murray, Michael T. *Natural Alternative to Over-the-Counter and Prescription Drugs.* New York: Morrow, 1994.

————. *Diabetes and Hypoglycemia: How You Can Benefit From Diet, Vitamins, Minerals, Herbs, Exercise and Other Natural Methods.* Rocklin, CA: Prima Publishing, 1994.

Ornstein, Robert, and David Sobel. *The Healing Brain.* New York: Simon & Schuster, 1988.

————. *Healthy Pleasures.* Reading, MA: Addison-Wesley, 1990.

Pelletier, Kenneth R. *Mind as Healer, Mind as Slayer.* Rev. ed. New York: Delacorte, 1992.

Reuben, Carolyn. *Antioxidants: Your Complete Guide.* Rocklin, CA: Prima Publishing, 1995.

Siegel, Bernie, M.D. *Love, Medicine and Miracles: Lessons Learned About Self-Healing From a Surgeon's Experience with Exceptional Patients.* Boston: G. K. Hall, 1988.

————. *Peace, Love and Healing: Bodymind Communication and the Path to Self-Healing.* New York: Harper & Row, 1989.

Weil, Andrew, M.D. *Spontaneous Healing.* Boston: Houghton Mifflin, 1994.

Weiner, Michael A. *Healing Children Naturally*. San Rafael, CA: Quantum Books, 1993.

Weiss, Brian, M.D. *Through Time into Healing*. New York: Simon & Schuster, 1992.

Nutrition/Supplementation

ADA's Nutrition Recommendations and Principles for People with Diabetes Mellitus. *Diabetes Care* 19, Suppl. 1 (1996): S18.

Balch, James F., and Phyllis Balch. *Prescription for Nutritional Healing*. Garden City Park, NY: Avery Publishing Group, 1993.

Ballentine, Rudolph. *Transition to Vegetarianism: An Evolutionary Step*. Honesdale, PA: Himalayan Publishers, 1987.

Colbin, Annemarie. *Food and Healing*. New York: Ballantine, 1986.

Gagne, Steve. *The Energetics of Food*. Santa Fe: Spiral Sciences, 1990.

Haas, Elson M., M.D. *Staying Healthy with Nutrition*. Berkeley: Celestial Arts, 1992.

Klaper, Michael, M.D. *Vegan Nutrition Pure and Simple*. Maui, Hawaii: Gentle World, 1987.

Lappe, Frances M. *Diet for a Small Planet*. Rev. ed. New York: Ballantine Books, 1975.

McDougall, John M., M.D. *McDougall's Medicine*. Piscataway, NJ: New Century, 1985.

McDougall, Mary. *The McDougall Health-Supporting Cookbook*. Clinton, NJ.: New Win Publishing, Volume I, 1985; Volume II, 1986.

McDougall, Mary. *The New McDougall Cookbook*. New York: Dutton, 1993.

Ohsawa, George. *The Art of Peace*. Oroville, CA: George Ohsawa Macrobiotic Foundation, 1990.

Pickarski, Ron. *Friendly Foods*. Berkeley: Ten Speed Press, 1991.

Pitchford, Paul. *Healing with Whole Foods: Oriental Traditions and Modern Nutrition*. Berkeley: North Atlantic Books, 1993.

The Pritikin Program for Diet and Exercise. New York: Grosset and Dunlap, 1979.

Robbins, John. *Diet for a New America: How Your Food Choices Affect Your Health, Happiness, and the Future of Life on Earth*. Walpole, NH: Stillpoint Publishing, 1987.

———. *May All Be Fed*. New York: Morrow, 1992; Avon, 1993.

Wasserman, Debbie. *Simply Vegan: Quick Vegetarian Meals*. Baltimore: Vegetarian Resource Group, 1991.

Werbach, Melvyn, M.D. *Healing with Food*. New York: HarperCollins, 1993.

White, J. R., and R. K. Campbell. Magnesium and diabetes: A review. *Ann Pharmacother* 27 (1993): 775–780.

Polarity Therapy

Beaulou, John. *Polarity Therapy Workbook*. New York: Bio Sonic Enterprises, 1994.

Stone, Randolph. *Health Building*. Sebastopol, Cal.: CRCS Publications, 1985.

Teschler, Wilfried. *The Polarity Healing Handbook*. Bath, England: Gateway Books, and San Leandro, California: Interbook, Inc., 1986.

Reflexology

Byers, Dwight. *Better Health with Foot Reflexology*. Available through the International Institute of Reflexology, P.O. Box 12642, St. Petersburg, FL 33733-2642.

Kunz, Kevin and Barbara Kunz. *Complete Guide to Foot Reflexology*. Rev. ed. Englewood Cliffs, NJ: Prentice-Hall, 1991.

———. *Hand and Foot Reflexology: A Self-Help Guide*. Englewood Cliffs, NJ: Prentice-Hall, 1984.

Norman, Laura. *Feet First: A Guide to Foot Reflexology*. New York: Simon & Schuster, 1988.

Wills, Pauline. *The Reflexology Manual: An Easy-to-Use Illustrated Guide to the Healing Zones of the Hands and Feet*. Rochester, VT: Healing Arts Press, 1995.

Tai Chi

Clark, Barbara. *Jin Shin Acutouch: The Tai Chi of Healing Arts*. San Diego: Clark Publishing, 1987.

Knocking at the Gate of Life and Other Healing Exercises From China. Translated by Edward C. Chang. Emmaus, PA.: Rodale Press, 1985.

Kuo, Simmone. *Long Life, Good Health through Tai-Chi Chuan*. Berkeley: North Atlantic Books, 1991.

Sutton, Nigel. *Applied Tai Chi Chuan*. London: A. & C. Black, 1991.

Yoga

Folan, Lilias. *Lilias, Yoga and Your Life*. New York: Macmillan, 1981.

Hewitt, James. *The Complete Yoga Book*. New York: Schocken Books, 1978.

Kundalini Research Institute. *Sadhana Guidelines for Kundalini Yoga Daily Practice*. Los Angeles: Arcline Publications, 1988.

Monro, Robin, et al. *Yoga for Common Ailments*. New York: Simon & Schuster, 1990.

Sivananda Yoga Vedanta Center. *Learn Yoga in a Weekend*. New York: Knopf, 1993.

Index

ABOUT THE AUTHOR

Deborah Mitchell is a medical writer and journalist specializing in natural medicine and nutrition topics. Her articles have appeared in consumer magazines and professional journals. She has ghostwritten or coauthored five books, including *The Good Sex Book: Recovering and Discovering Your Sexual Self, The Natural Health Guide to Headache Relief,* and *Natural Medicine for Back Pain.* She is currently working on two books for the Dell Natural Medicine series. Deborah lives and works in Tucson, Arizona.